MW00988173

Other books in this series include:

Curing Insomnia Naturally with Chinese Medicine

Curing Hay Fever Naturally with Chinese Medicine

Breast Health Naturally with Chinese Medicine

Curing Depression Naturally with Chinese Medicine

Curing Arthritis Naturally with Chinese Medicine

Curing PMS Naturally with Chinese Medicine

Curing Headaches Naturally

with Chinese Medicine

Bob Flaws

BLUE POPPY PRESS

Published by:
BLUE POPPY PRESS, INC.
3450 Penrose Place, Suite 110
BOULDER, CO 80301

First Edition, October, 1998
ISBN 0-936185-95-3 LC 98-71000
COPYRIGHT 1998 © BLUE POPPY PRESS

WARNING: When following some of the self-care techniques given in this book, failure to follow the author's instruction may result in side effects or negative reactions. Therefore, please be sure to follow the author's instructions carefully for all self-care techniques and modalities. For instance, wrong or excessive application of moxibustion may cause local burns with redness, inflammation, blistering, or even possible scarring. If you have any questions about doing these techniques safely and without unwanted side effects, please see a local professional practitioner for instruction.

DISCLAIMER: The information in this book is given in good faith. However, the author and the publishers cannot be held responsible for any error or omission. The publishers will not accept liabilities for any injuries or damages caused to the reader that may result from the reader's acting upon or using the content contained in this book.

COMP Designation: Original work and functionally translated compilation

Printed at Johnson Printing in Boulder, CO
on essentially chlorine-free paper
Cover design by Jeff Fuller, Crescent Moon
10 9 8 7 6 5 4 3 2 1

Preface

Several years ago, I wrote a book called *Migraines and Traditional Chinese Medicine: A Layperson's Guide*. Although that book sold quite well, eventually it no longer represented the state of my art and it was allowed to go out of print. When Blue Poppy Press decided to do a whole new series of layperson's books on various diseases and Chinese medicine, everyone said that I *had* to rewrite *Migraines* to fit this series. However, *Migraines* was only about that particular kind of headache, and I felt that a more general book on all sorts of headaches would be more useful to more readers.

Therefore, the following book is a layperson's introduction to Chinese medicine and headaches. It covers the Chinese theories about what causes headaches as well as the diagnosis and treatment of headaches with acupuncture and Chinese herbal medicine. In addition, it includes a host of low or no cost home remedies to both prevent and treat headaches. These remedies include Chinese dietary therapy, Chinese self-massage, Chinese herbal teas, wines, and porridges, moxibustion, aromatherapy, herbal inhalants, hydrotherapy, and poultices and plasters.

Based on my 20 years of clinical experience and as an occasional migraine sufferer myself, I believe that Chinese medicine is extremely effective for curing, not just relieving, the majority of chronic, recurrent headaches. Not only can it relieve the localized pain and pressure, but, because it treats by returning the entire organis to a harmonious state of balance, patients typically report that they are generally healthier and well.

Chinese medicine is a rising star in the realm of alternative or complementary health in the world today, and rightly so! As the oldest, continually practiced, literate, professional medicine in the world, Chinese medicine is a vast treasure house filled with wise theories and compassionate treatments. Therefore, I have written this book in the hope that more Westerners try Chinese medicine and see what it can do for them.

Bob Flaws
Boulder, CO
Nov. 1997

Table of Contents

Introduction

Jean has secreted herself in her bedroom, door closed, lights off, and the curtains tightly shut. The left side of her head is pounding, she is sick to her stomach, and she cannot stand any noise or light. Two hours before, she had felt a familiar numb sensation on the side of her mouth followed by tingling in her hands and a narrowing of her field of vision. When she felt these sensations, she knew she was in for another one of her "killer" migraines. For several hours she will be in agony. Eventually, she will vomit and have diarrhea. After that, she will fall asleep. When she wakes up the next morning, she will feel as if she had been through a wringer, but at least she can go back to work. This same scenario plays itself out several times per year. Over-the-counter Western headache medicine doesn't touch Jean's pain, and she is afraid to use Western prescription drugs.

In the case above, Jean is having a pretty severe migraine headache. Your headaches may not be so severe. Perhaps yours is more of a tension headache. However, no matter what kind of headache you suffer from, Chinese medicine can probably help you either eliminate headaches altogether or, at the least, minimize their frequency and severity. Chinese doctors have been treating all kinds of headaches for not less than 2,000 recorded years. During that time, 100 generations of highly trained, literate professional practitioners have written down their experiences in treating headaches with acupuncture, Chinese herbal medicine, and a number of other Asian treatment methods. In addition, hundreds of research studies have been conducted since 1949 in the People's Republic of China on the

Chinese medical treatment of this all too common complaint. Therefore, that Chinese medicine does treat headaches very well is a well-established fact.

Some Western information on headaches

However, before we jump into the Chinese medical description of the causes and treatment of headache, it is useful to first introduce a little basic information on what Western medicine has to say about headaches. After all, this book has been written mainly for people living in the Western world.

The two most common types of headaches according to Western medicine are tension headaches and migraines.[1] The symptoms of tension headaches are a dull, steady, non-throbbing pain usually felt on both sides of the head. This pain may be either mild or severe. Sometimes, your head may feel like it is in the grip of a vise or that your head is being squeezed by a tight band. Commonly, the pain extends to the neck and shoulders. Such tension headaches may last 1-2 hours or all day. They often occur in the late afternoon or evening as a result of accumulated stress during the day. Some people may have chronic tension headaches which occur on a daily or almost daily basis and this may go on for months and even years. According to Western medicine, the causes of this kind of tension headache are emotional stress resulting in tightening of the muscles of the head and neck. However, tension headaches may also be caused by poor posture, remaining in the same position for too long, or arthritis.

Migraine headaches, on the other hand, are characterized by moderate to severe pounding or throbbing pain mostly commonly felt on only one side of the head. Often, these one-sided headaches are accompanied by nausea, vomiting, dizziness, and

---

[1] "Get a Handle on Your Headache Type", Excedrin Headache Resource Center, http://www.excedrin.com/excedrin/workbook1.html

hypersensitivity to light and/or sound. About 10-15% of migraine sufferers experience an "aura" or "prodrome" before the pain in their heads begins. Such auras include visual disturbances, such as flashing spots, colors, lines, or shapes, or temporary reductions in their field of vision, such as tunnel vision. When head pain is preceded by such distortions in vision, this is called a classic migraine, while so-called common migraines are not preceded by any visual auras. Although as much as 25% of the population probably experience a migrainous attack at least once in their life, 70% of migraine sufferers are women. Migraines may last from a few hours to three days and may come only a couple of times in a life or several times a week. The average number of attacks is 1-3 times per month and attacks often correspond to certain times in the menstrual cycle in women. Ninety percent of migraine sufferers have a close relative who also has/had migraines.

In terms of what triggers migraines in those who are predisposed to get them, certain foods, such as nuts, cheeses, avocados, chocolate, bacon, ham, hot dogs and cold cuts, alcohol, caffeine, changes in weather or sleep patterns, skipped meals, some medications, and stress all play a part to varying degrees in different individuals. Bright lights, cigarette smoke, intense heat, or loud noises can also precipitate an attack in some people. Further, there is a link between oral birth control pills and hormone replacement therapy in menopausal women and migraines.

Besides these two main types of headaches, there are several others worth noting, since one of these other types may be the kind of headache you suffer from. Cluster headaches are relatively uncommon but, when they occur, they cause excruciating, knife-like pain around or "in" one eye. They are called cluster headaches because sufferers typically will have an attack every day, usually at the same time each day, for several weeks or months. Then they disappear for months or even years. Ninety percent of cluster headache patients are men.

Rebound headaches occur in patients who have overused headache medications due to persistent headache pain. In this case, the headache medicine which was taken to get rid of the pain actually turns around and makes the headache worse.

Sinus headaches refer to pain in the head and face regions due to pressure from mucus build-up in the sinuses in turn due to infection. The patient typically has a green, pussy nasal discharge, nasal congestion, and tenderness over the affected sinus. Typically, this pain is worse in the morning and worse in cold, damp weather. There is commonly a recent history of cold or hayfever. Many people who think they have "sinus" headaches, actually have tension or migraine headaches.

East is East & West is West

Chinese medicine is a distinct and separate system of medical thought and practice from modern Western medicine. This means that one must shift models of reality when it comes to thinking about Chinese medicine. It has taken the Chinese more than 2,000 years to develop this medical system. Having spent the last 20 years of my life both practicing Chinese medicine in the West and writing and teaching about it, I feel very strongly that one cannot understand Chinese medicine by trying to explain it in Western scientific or medical terms.

Most people reading this book have probably taken high school biology back when they were sophomores. Whether we recognize it or not, most of us Westerners think of what we learned about the human body in high school as "the really real" description of reality, not one possible description. However, if Chinese medicine is to make any sense to Westerners at all, one must be able to entertain the notion that there are potentially other valid descriptions of the human body, its functions, health, and disease. In grappling with this fundamentally important issue, it is useful to think about the concepts of a map and the terrain it describes.

If we take the United States of America as an example, we can have numerous different maps of this country's land mass. One map might show population. Another might show per capita incomes. Another might show religious or ethnic distributions. Yet another might be a road map. And still another might be a map showing political, *i.e.*, state boundaries. In fact, there could

5

be an infinite number of potentially different maps of the United States depending on what one was trying to show and do. As long as the map is based on accurate information and has been created with self-consistent logic, then one map is not necessarily more correct than another. The issue is to use the right map for what you are trying to do. If one wants to drive from Chicago to Washington, D.C., then a road map is probably the right one *for that job* but is not necessarily a truer or "more real" description of the United States than a map showing annual rainfall.

What I am getting at here is that *the map is not the terrain*. The Western biological map of the human body is only one potentially useful medical map. It is no more true than the traditional Chinese medical map, and the "facts" of one map cannot be reduced to the criteria or standards of another *unless they share the same logic right from the beginning*. As long as the Western medical map is capable of solving a person's disease in a cost-effective, time-efficient manner without side effects or iatrogenesis (meaning doctor-caused disease), then it is a useful map. Chinese medicine needs to be judged in the same way. The Chinese medical map of health and disease is just as "real" as the Western biological map as long as, using it, professional practitioners and their patients are able to solve their patients' health problems in a safe and effective way.

Therefore, the following chapter is an introduction to the basics of Chinese medicine. Unless one understands some of the fundamental theories and "facts" of Chinese medicine, one will not be able to understand or accept the reasons for some of the Chinese medical treatments of headaches. As the reader will quickly see from this brief overview of Chinese medicine, "This doesn't look like Kansas, Toto!"

An Overview of the Chinese Medical Map

In this chapter, we will look at an overview of Chinese medicine. In particular, we will discuss yin and yang, qi and blood, essence and spirit, the viscera and bowels, and the channels and network vessels. In the following chapter, we will look at the concept of pain in Chinese medicine. Once we understand these things , we can then go on to see how Chinese medicine views headaches and how professional practitioners of Chinese medicine diagnose and treat various patterns of headache.

Yin & Yang

To understand Chinese medicine, one must first understand the concepts of yin and yang since these are the most basic concepts in this system. Yin and yang are the cornerstones for understanding, diagnosing, and treating the body and mind in Chinese medicine. In a sense, all the other theories and concepts of Chinese medicine are nothing other than an elaboration of yin and yang. Most people have probably already heard of yin and yang but may have only a fuzzy idea of what these terms mean.

The concepts of yin and yang can be used to describe everything that exists in the universe, including all the parts and functions of the body. Originally, yin referred to the shady side of a hill and yang to the sunny side of the hill. Since sunshine and shade are two, interdependent sides of a single reality, these two aspects of the hill are seen as part of a single whole. Other examples of yin and yang are that night exists only in relation to day and cold exists only in relation to heat. According to Chinese thought, every single thing that exists in the universe has these two aspects, a yin and a yang. Thus everything has a front and a back, a top and a bottom, a left and a right, and a beginning and an end. However, a thing is yin or yang *only in relation to its paired complement*. Nothing is in itself yin or yang.

It is the concepts of yin and yang which make Chinese medicine a holistic medicine. This is because, based on this unitary and complementary vision of reality, no body part or body function is viewed as separate or isolated from the whole person. The table below shows a partial list of yin and yang pairs as they apply to

Yin	Yang
form	function
viscera	bowels
blood	qi
inside	outside
front of body	back of body
right side	left side
lower body	upper body
cool, cold	warm, hot
stillness	activity, movement

the body. However, it is important to remember that each item listed is either yin or yang only in relation to its complementary partner. Nothing is absolutely and all by itself either yin or yang. As we can see from the above list, it is possible to describe every aspect of the body in terms of yin and yang.

Qi

Qi (pronounced chee) and blood are the two most important complementary pairs of yin and yang within the human body. It is said that, in the world, yin and yang are water and fire, but in the human body, yin and yang are blood and qi. Qi is yang in relation to blood which is yin. Qi is often translated as energy and certainly energy is a manifestation of qi. Chinese language scholars would say, however, that qi is larger than any single type of energy described by modern Western science. Paul Unschuld, perhaps the greatest living sinologist, translates the word qi as influences. This conveys the sense that qi is what is responsible for change and movement. Thus, within Chinese medicine, qi is that which motivates all movement and transformation or change.

In Chinese medicine, qi is defined as having five specific functions:

1. Defense
It is qi which is responsible for protecting the exterior of the body from invasion by external pathogens. This qi, called defensive qi, flows through the exterior portion of the body.

2. Transformation
Qi transforms substances so that they can be utilized by the body. An example of this function is the transformation of the food we eat into nutrients to nourish the body, thus producing more qi and blood.

3. Warming
Qi, being relatively yang, is inherently warm and one of the main functions of the qi is to warm the entire body, both inside and out. If this warming function of the qi is weak, cold may cause the flow of qi and blood to be congealed similar to cold's effect on water producing ice.

4. Restraint

It is qi which holds all the organs and substances in their proper place. Thus all the organs, blood, and fluids need qi to keep them from falling or leaking out of their specific pathways. If this function of the qi is weak, then problems like uterine prolapse, easy bruising, or urinary incontinence may occur.

5. Transportation

Qi provides the motivating force for all transportation and movement in the body. Every aspect of the body that moves is moved by the qi. Hence the qi moves the blood and body fluids throughout the body. It moves food through the stomach and blood through the vessels.

Blood

In Chinese medicine, blood refers to the red fluid that flows through our vessels the same as in modern Western medicine, but it also has meanings and implications which are different from those in modern Western medicine. Most basically, blood is that substance which nourishes and moistens all the body tissues. Without blood, no body tissue can function properly. In addition, when blood is insufficient or scanty, tissue becomes dry and withers.

Qi and blood are closely interrelated. It is said that, "Qi is the commander of the blood and blood is the mother of qi." This means that it is qi which moves the blood but that it is the blood which provides the nourishment and physical foundation for the creation and existence of the qi.

In Chinese medicine, blood provides the following functions for the body:

1. Nourishment

Blood nourishes the body. Along with qi, the blood goes to every part of the body. When the blood is insufficient, function decreases and tissue atrophies or shrinks.

10

2. Moistening

Blood moistens the body tissues. This includes the skin, eyes, and ligaments and tendons or what are simply called the sinews of body in Chinese medicine. Thus blood insufficiency can cause drying out and consequent stiffening of various body tissues throughout the body.

3. Blood provides the material foundation for the spirit or mind.

In Chinese medicine, the mind and body are not two separate things. The spirit is nothing other than a great accumulation of qi. The blood (yin) supplies the material support and nourishment for the spirit (yang) so that it accumulates, becomes bright (*i.e.*, conscious and clever), and stays rooted in the body. If the blood becomes insufficient, the mind can "float," causing problems like insomnia, agitation, and unrest.

Essence

Along with qi and blood, essence is one of the three most important constituents of the body. Essence is the most fundamental, essential material the body utilizes for its growth, maturation, and reproduction. There are two forms of this essence. We inherit essence from our parents and we also produce our own essence from the food we eat, the liquids we drink, and the air we breathe.

The essence which comes from our parents is what determines our basic constitution, strength, and vitality. We each have a finite, limited amount of this inherited essence. It is important to protect and conserve this essence because all bodily functions depend upon it, and, when it is gone, we die. Thus the depletion of essence has serious implications for our overall health and well-being. Happily, the essence derived from food and drink helps to bolster and support this inherited essence. Thus, if we eat well and do not consume more qi and blood than we create each day, then when we sleep at night, this surplus qi and more especially blood is transformed into essence.

11

It is said in Chinese medicine that essence is stored in the kidneys. But the place where the kidneys store this essence is not necessarily in the kidneys themselves but may also be in other tissues associated with the kidneys. For instance, it is said that stored essence becomes the marrow. Marrow in Chinese medicine means the bone marrow but also the nerves found in the spine, while the brain is called the sea of marrow. We will see below that essence plays an important role in at least one kind of headache based on the fact that, "The brain is the sea of marrow."

Spirit

Spirit in Chinese medicine means one's mental-emotional faculties. Basically, it is a way of saying consciousness. In Chinese medicine, this term does not have any religious or "spiritual" connotation. Spirit in a Chinese medical sense is nothing other than the accumulation of qi and blood in the heart. If enough qi and blood accumulates in the heart, then this gives rise to consciousness which in Chinese medicine is called the spirit. Because of the interrelationship between the essence, the qi, and the spirit, sometimes consciousness is called the "essence spirit." If one is particularly talking about the emotions, then the compound term "spirit will" (will meaning desire) is commonly used. At other times, because the spirit is associated with mental clarity, the compound term "spirit brightness" or "spirit brilliance" is used. In order for there to be spirit, there must be sufficient qi. But in order for that spirit to be calm and healthy, there must be sufficient blood to nourish the spirit and keep it under control. Because the spirit made from qi is inherently yang in nature, it tends to stir or become restless if yin blood does not nourish and "mother" it. Therefore, normal mental clarity is referred to as "having spirit", while emotional upsetment is referred to as "spirit not quiet" or "restless spirit."

On the one hand, the spirit is made up from the qi and blood which are produced by the viscera and bowels we will talk about

12

next. On the other, the qi and, therefore, the spirit are affected by external stimuli. Thus, there is no dichotomy or division in Chinese medicine between the psychological and biological. The mind arises as a function of the viscera and bowels, but the functioning of the viscera and bowels is affected by the experiences of the mind and emotions. In fact, every thought in the mind or felt emotion is nothing other than the experience of the movement of qi. If one changes the way the qi moves, one changes one's mental-emotional experience, while changing one's mind and emotions changes the way the qi moves. Hence the qi and the spirit or mind are not two different things but rather a single reality.

The Viscera & Bowels

In Chinese medicine, the internal organs (called viscera so as not to become confused with the Western biological entities of the same name) have a wider area of function and influence than in Western medicine. Each viscus has distinct responsibilities for maintaining the physical and psychological health of the individual. When thinking about the internal viscera according to Chinese medicine, it is more accurate to view them as spheres of influence or a network that spreads throughout the body, rather than as a distinct and separate physical organ as described by Western science. This is why the famous German sinologist, Manfred Porkert, refers to them as orbs rather than as organs. In Chinese medicine, the relationship between the various viscera and other parts of the body is made possible by the channel and network vessel system which we will discuss below.

In Chinese medicine, there are five main viscera which are relatively yin and six main bowels which are relatively yang. The five yin viscera are the heart, lungs, liver, spleen, and kidneys. The six yang bowels are the stomach, small intestine, large intestine, gallbladder, urinary bladder, and a system that Chinese medicine refers to as the triple burner. All the functions of the entire body are subsumed or described under these eleven organs or spheres of influence. Thus Chinese medicine *as a system* does not have a pancreas, a pituitary gland, or the ovaries. Nonetheless, all the functions of these Western organs are described under the Chinese medical system of the five viscera and six bowels.

Visceral Correspondences

Organ	Tissue	Sense	Emotion
Kidneys	bones/ head hair	hearing	fear
Liver	sinews	sight	anger
Spleen	flesh	taste	thinking/ worry
Lungs	skin/body hair	smell	grief/ sadness
Heart	blood vessels	speech	joy/fright

Within this system, the five viscera are the most important. These are the organs that Chinese medicine says are responsible for the creation and transformation of qi and blood and the storage of essence. For instance, the kidneys are responsible for the excretion of urine but are also responsible for hearing, the strength of the bones, sex, reproduction, maturation and growth, the lower and upper back, and the lower legs in general and the knees in particular. This points out that the Chinese viscera may have the same name and even some overlapping functions but yet are quite different from the organs of modern Western medicine. Each of the five Chinese medical viscera also has a corresponding tissue, sense, and emotion related to it. These are outlined in the table above.

In addition, each Chinese medical viscus or bowel possesses both a yin and a yang aspect. The yin aspect of a viscus or bowel refers to its substantial nature or tangible form. Further, an organ's yin is responsible for the nurturing, cooling, and moistening of that viscus or bowel. The yang aspect of the viscus or bowel represents its functional activities or what it does. An organ's yang aspect is also warming. These two aspects, yin and yang, form and function, cooling and heating, when balanced create good health. However, if either yin or yang becomes too strong or too weak, the result will be disease.

Four out of five of the viscera are potentially associated with the causes and mechanisms of headaches. These include the liver, spleen, heart, and kidneys. Only two of the six bowels are associated with headaches in Chinese medicine—the gallbladder and stomach. Below are the main statements of fact in Chinese medicine regarding these four viscera and two bowels which we will be using in our description of the diagnosis and treatment of headaches. For a more complete listing of the statements of fact pertaining to all the five viscera and six bowels, see my *Statements of Fact in Traditional Chinese Medicine* also published by Blue Poppy Press.

The kidneys

In Chinese medicine, the kidneys are considered to be the foundation of our life. Because the developing fetus looks like a large kidney and because the kidneys are the main viscus for the storage of inherited essence, the kidneys are referred to as the prenatal root. Thus keeping the kidney qi strong and kidney yin and yang in relative balance is considered essential to good health and longevity. Some basic Chinese medical statements of fact about the kidneys which are relevant to the mechanisms of depression are:

1. The kidneys are considered responsible for human reproduction, development, and maturation.
These are the same functions we used when describing the essence. This is because the essence is stored in the kidneys. Health problems related to reproduction, development, and maturation are considered to be problems of the kidney essence. Excessive sexual activity, drug use, or simple prolonged over-exhaustion can all damage and consume kidney essence. Kidney essence is also consumed by the simple act of aging.

2. The kidneys are the foundation of water metabolism.
The kidneys work in coordination with the lungs and spleen to insure that water is spread properly throughout the body and that excess water is excreted as urination. Therefore, problems such as edema, excessive dryness, or excessive day or nighttime urination can indicate a weakness of kidney function.

3. The kidneys store the will.
Will here means desire. If kidney qi is insufficient, this aspect of our human nature can be weakened. Conversely, pushing ourselves to extremes, such as long distance running or cycling, can eventually exhaust our kidneys.

4. Fear is the emotion associated with the kidneys.
This means that fear can manifest when the kidney qi is insufficient. Vice versa, constant or excessive fear can damage the kidneys and make them weak.

5. The kidneys govern the bones. The bones engender the marrow. The brain is the sea of marrow.
This means that there is a very close relationship between kidney essence and the brain. If kidney essence becomes insufficient, the brain may lose its nourishment and filling.

6. The low back is the mansion of the kidneys.
If the kidneys become weak and vacuous, then low back pain is one of the key symptoms of this.

7. Kidney water moistens liver wood.
The kidneys are the "mother" of the liver. In particular, it is kidney yin or kidney water which moistens and enriches the liver, keeping the liver soft and harmonious.

The liver

In Chinese medicine, the liver is associated with one's emotional state, with digestion, and with menstruation in women. The basic Chinese medical statements of fact concerning the liver include:

1. The liver controls coursing and discharge.
Coursing and discharge refer to the uninhibited spreading of qi to every part of the body. If the liver is not able to maintain the free and smooth flow of qi throughout the body, multiple physical and emotional symptoms can develop. This function of the liver is most easily damaged by emotional causes and, in particular, by anger and frustration. For example, if the liver is stressed due to pent-up anger, the flow of liver qi can become depressed or stagnate.

Liver qi stagnation can cause a wide range of health problems, including PMS, chronic digestive disturbance, depression, and insomnia. Therefore, it is essential to keep our liver qi flowing freely.

2. The liver stores the blood.
This means that the liver regulates the amount of blood in circulation. In particular, when the body is at rest, the blood in the extremities returns to the liver. As an extension of this, it is said in Chinese medicine that the liver is yin in form but yang in function. Thus the liver requires sufficient blood to keep it and its associated tissues moist and supple, cool and relaxed.

3. The emotion associated with the liver is anger.
Anger is the emotion that typically arises when the liver is diseased and especially when its qi does not flow freely.

17

Conversely, anger damages the liver. Thus the emotions related to the stagnation of qi in the liver are frustration, anger, and rage.

4. The liver governs upbearing and effusion.
As long as the liver courses and discharges the qi, the qi moves upward and outward in a healthy and harmonious way. However, if the liver qi becomes depressed and stagnant, it may eventually vent itself upward in the body (upward due to its yang nature) in a pathological way. Therefore, most erroneous upward counterflow of qi is associated with the liver in Chinese medicine. As we will see below, pathological upward counterflow of qi to the head is a main cause of headaches.

The heart

The heart's role in the cause and mechanisms of headaches primarily revolves around the heart's role in the creation and control of blood. The basic statements of fact about the heart in Chinese medicine which relate to the blood are:

1. The heart governs the blood.
This means that it is the heart qi which "stirs" or moves the blood within its vessels. This is roughly analogous to the heart's pumping the blood in Western medicine. The pulsation of the blood through the arteries due to the contraction of the heart is referred to as the "stirring of the pulse." In fact, the Chinese word for pulse and vessel is the same. So this could also be translated as the "stirring of the vessels."

2. The heart stores the spirit.
The spirit refers to the mind in Chinese medicine. Therefore, this statement underscores that mental function, mental clarity, and mental equilibrium are all associated with the heart. If the heart does not receive enough qi or blood or if the heart is disturbed by something, the spirit may become restless and this may produce

symptoms of mental-emotional unrest, heart palpitations, insomnia, profuse dreams, etc.

3. The heart governs the vessels.
This statement is very close to number one above. The vessels refer to the blood vessels and also to the pulse.

The spleen

The spleen is less important in Western medicine than it is in Chinese medicine. Since at least the Yuan dynasty (1280-1368 CE), the spleen has been one of the two most important viscera of Chinese medicine (the other being the kidneys). In Chinese medicine, the spleen plays a pivotal role in the creation of qi and blood and in the circulation and transformation of body fluids. Therefore, when it comes to the spleen, it is especially important not to think of this Chinese viscus in the same way as the Western spleen. The main statements of fact concerning the spleen in Chinese medicine, which help explain headaches are:

1. The spleen governs movement and transformation.
This refers to the movement and transformation of foods and liquids through the digestive system. In this case, movement and transformation may be paraphrased as digestion. However, secondarily, movement and transformation also refer to the movement and transformation of body fluids through the body. It is the spleen qi which is largely responsible for controlling liquid metabolism in the body.

2. The spleen restrains the blood.
As mentioned above, one of the five functions of the qi is to restrain the fluids of the body, including the blood, within their proper channels and reservoirs. If the spleen qi is healthy and abundant, then the blood is held within its vessels properly. However, if the spleen qi becomes weak and insufficient, then the blood may flow outside its channels and vessels resulting in various types of pathological bleeding. This includes various

19

types of pathological bleeding associated with the menstrual cycle.

3. The spleen stores the constructive.
The constructive is one of the types of qi in the body. Specifically, it is the qi responsible for nourishing and constructing the body and its tissues. This constructive qi is closely associated with the process of digestion and the creation of qi and blood out of food and liquids. If the spleen fails to store or runs out of constructive qi, then the person becomes hungry on the one hand, and eventually becomes fatigued on the other.

4. Thought is the emotion associated with the spleen.
In the West, we do not usually think of thought as an emotion per se. Be that as it may, in Chinese medicine it is classified along with anger, joy, fear, grief, and melancholy. In particular, thinking, or perhaps I should say over-thinking, causes the spleen qi to bind. This means that the spleen qi does not flow harmoniously and this typically manifests as loss of appetite, abdominal bloating after meals, and indigestion.

5. The spleen is the source of engenderment and transformation.
Engenderment and transformation refer to the creation or production of the qi and blood out of the food and drink we take in each day. If the spleen receives adequate food and drink and then properly transforms that food and drink, it engenders or creates the qi and blood. Although the kidneys and lungs also participate in the creation of the qi, while the kidneys and heart also participate in the creation of the blood, the spleen is the pivotal viscus in both processes, and spleen qi weakness and insufficiency is a leading cause of qi and blood insufficiency and weakness.

The gallbladder

The main statements of fact concerning the gallbladder in terms of headaches in Chinese medicine are:

1. The gallbladder governs decision.

In Chinese medicine, the liver is likened to a general who plans strategy for the body, while the gallbladder is likened to a judge. According to this point of view, if a person lacks gallbladder qi, they will have trouble making decisions. In addition, they will be timid. While courage in the West is associated with the heart (*coeur* = courage), bravery in the East is associated with the gallbladder. Actually, this is also an old Western idea as well. When someone is very forward and brazen, we say that "They have gall." Conversely, if someone is excessively timid, this may be due to gallbladder qi vacuity or insufficiency.

2. The liver and gallbladder have the same palace.

This statement underscores the particularly close relationship between the liver and gallbladder. If the liver becomes diseased, this often manifests along the pathways of the gallbladder channel.

The stomach

There are a number of important statements of fact concerning the stomach in Chinese medicine due to the stomach's pivotal role in digestion and , therefore, in the creation of qi and blood. Below we will only discuss those statements which we will use later in our discussion of the disease causes and disease mechanisms of headache in Chinese medicine.

1. The stomach governs intake.

This means that the stomach is the first to receive foods and drinks ingested into the body.

2. The stomach governs downbearing of the turbid.

The process of digestion in Chinese medicine is likened to the process of fermentation and then distillation. The stomach is the fermentation tun wherein foods and liquids are "rotted and ripened." This rottening and ripening allows for the separation of clear and turbid parts of the digestate. The spleen sends the

21

clear parts upward to the lungs and heart to become the qi and blood respectively. The stomach's job is to send the turbid part down to be excreted as waste from the large intestine and bladder.

3. Stomach likes harmony and downbearing.
The normal movement of the stomach's qi is downward. If the stomach becomes diseased, its qi frequently counterflows upward. This results in nausea and vomiting. If liver qi counterflows upward, this can easily draft the stomach qi upward along with it. Another statement which is an extension of this goes, "The stomach is the central pivot for the upbearing and downbearing of yin and yang." Any disease affecting the stomach may affect normal upbearing and downbearing, while any disease of the stomach may affect the upbearing and downbearing of the rest of the body.

Above we mentioned that there are five viscera and six bowels. The sixth bowel is called the triple burner. It is said in Chinese medicine that, "The triple burner has a function but no form." The name triple burner refers to the three main areas of the torso. The upper burner is the chest. The middle burner is the space from the bottom of the rib-cage to the level of the navel. The lower burner is the lower abdomen below the navel. These three spaces are called burners because all of the functions and transformations of the viscera and bowels which they contain are "warm" transformations similar to food cooking in a pot on a stove or similar to an alchemical transformation in a furnace. In fact, the triple burner is nothing other than a generalized concept of how the other viscera and bowels function together as an organic unit in terms of the digestion of foods and liquids and the circulation and transformation of body fluids.

The Channels & Network Vessels

Each viscus and bowel has a corresponding channel with which it is connected. In Chinese medicine, the inside of the body is made up of the viscera and bowels. The outside of the body is composed of the sinews and bones, muscles and flesh, and skin and hair. It is the channels and network vessels (*i.e.*, smaller connecting vessels) which connect the inside and the outside of the body. It is through these channels and network vessels that the viscera and bowels connect with their corresponding body tissues.

The channels and network vessel system is a unique feature of traditional Chinese medicine. These channels and vessels are different from the circulatory, nervous, or lymphatic systems. The earliest reference to these channels and vessels is in *Nei Jing (Inner Classic)*, a text written around the 2nd or 3rd century BCE.

The channels and vessels perform two basic functions. They are the pathways by which the qi and blood circulate through the body and between the organs and tissues. Additionally, as mentioned above, the channels connect the viscera and bowels internally with the exterior part of the body. This channel and vessel system functions in the body much like the world information communication network. The channels allow the various parts of our body to cooperate and interact to maintain our lives.

This channel and network vessel system is complex. There are 12 primary channels, six yin and six yang, each with a specific pathway through the external body and connected with an internal organ (see diagram below). There are also extraordinary vessels, sinew channels, channel divergences, main network vessels, and ultimately countless finer and finer network vessels permeating the entire body. All of these form a closed loop or circuit similar to but distinct from the Western circulatory system.

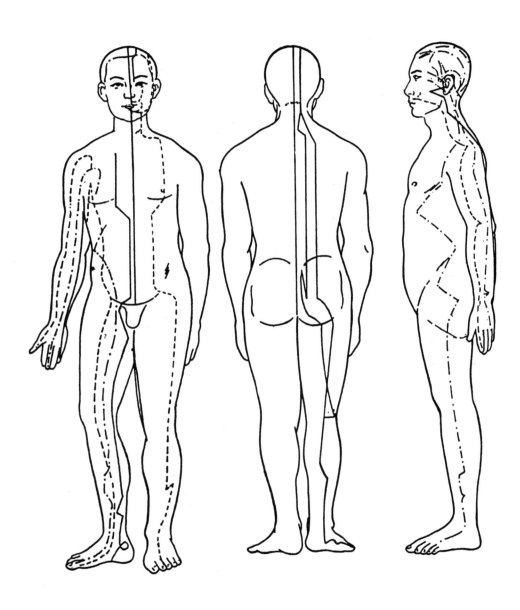

Acupuncture points are places located on the major channels where there is a special concentration of qi and blood. Because of the relatively more qi and blood accumulated at these places, the sites act as switches which can potentially control the flow of qi and blood in the channel on which the point is located. By stimulating these points in any of a number of different ways, one can speed up or slow down, make more or reduce, warm or cool down the qi and blood flowing in the channels and vessels. The main ways of stimulating these points and thus adjusting the flow of qi and blood in the channels and vessels is to needle them and to heat them by moxibustion.[2] Other commonly used ways of stimulating these points and thus adjusting the qi and blood flowing through the channels and vessels are massage, cupping, the application of magnets, and the application of various herbal medicinals. If the channels and vessels are the pathways over which the qi and blood flow, then the acupuncture points are the places where this flow can be adjusted.

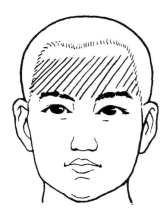

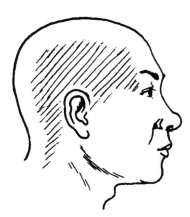

Yang Ming Area   *Shao Yang* Area

---

2   Moxibustion refers to adding heat to an acupuncture point or area of the body by burning a dried herb, Folium Artemisae Argyii (*Ai Ye*), Oriental mugwort, on, over, or near the area to be warmed.

25

The area of the head is divided into four general regions in terms of Chinese channels. The forehead and front of the face is the area traversed by the *yang ming* channels. The *yang ming* means the large intestine and stomach channels. The sides of the head is the area traversed by the *shao yang* channels. The *shao yang* means the gallbladder and triple burner channels. The back of the head is the area traversed by the *tai yang*. The *tai yang* means the bladder and small intestine channels. However, both these channels connect with the governing vessel which is also usually involved in back of the head headaches. The top of the head is where an internal branch of the *jue yin* ends. The *jue yin* in terms of headache means the liver channel.

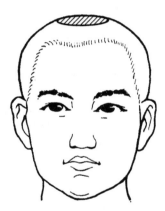
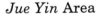
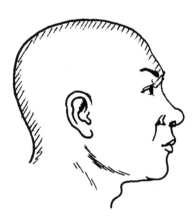

Jue Yin Area   *Tai Yang* Area

Pain in Chinese Medicine

There is a basic dictum in Chinese medicine about pain. This saying covers all types of pain felt anywhere in the body for any reason. The saying goes, "If there is pain, there is no free flow; if there is free flow, there is no pain." In other words, pain is the body's immediate felt sensation of a lack of free flow of the qi, blood, and body fluids. As long as the qi, blood, and body fluids are freely and smoothly flowing, there is no pain.

Lack of free flow can be due to either of two basic causes—either something is blocking and obstructing free flow or there is not sufficient qi or blood to flow freely. These are the only two broad categories of lack of free flow. Therefore, they are also the only two fundamental causes of all pain felt anywhere in the body. It does not matter whether the pain is strong or weak, instantaneous or lingering, sharp or dull, localized or moves about; there are only these two main reasons for pain in Chinese medicine.

Blockage & obstruction

Internal causes
The first main cause of lack of free flow and, therefore pain is blockage and obstruction. In other words, there is sufficient qi and blood to flow freely, but something has become stagnant and gathered. Thus the qi and blood flow is hindered and blocked. There are six things which may become blocked and inhibit free flow in the body. These are referred to as the six depressions. They are qi, blood, dampness, phlegm, food, and fire.

As we have already seen, if the liver loses its control over coursing and discharging, the qi will not spread freely throughout the body. Rather, it stagnates and accumulates. This is mostly due to what in Chinese is referred to as, "The emotions not being fulfilled." The implication of this is that all our emotions, which are merely the subjective feelings associated with various desires, put the qi in motion. If the desire is fulfilled, the qi can run its course. If the desire cannot be fulfilled, the movement of qi towards or away from the object of its desire is thwarted. This thwarting of one's desires or emotions causes the liver to lose its function and the qi to become stagnant and depressed. Thus the qi fails to flow freely, and this can cause pain.

In Chinese medicine, it is said that, "The qi moves the blood. If the qi moves, the blood moves. If the qi stops, the blood stops." If there is liver depression qi stagnation due to emotional stress and frustration, then, over time, this will also lead to blood stasis. Static blood is also a lack of free flow. Therefore, static blood or blood stasis is another cause of pain. Static blood may also be directly caused by traumatic injury. If static blood due to traumatic injury is not dispelled, it will also impede the flow of qi, since both the qi and blood flow together. In that case, static blood, which is yin and substantial, impedes the free flow of yang qi which is insubstantial and cannot penetrate the accumulated static blood.

Just as qi and blood flow together and form a yin-yang pair, body fluids also flow through the body and have a reciprocal relationship with both the qi and blood. The qi moves and transforms body fluids. If the qi becomes stagnant, then body fluids may also accumulate, just as the blood becomes static. If body fluids accumulate pathologically and are not moved and transformed, these are referred to as damp depression. Conversely, if for any other reason, dampness is formed, it may hinder and obstruct the free flow of qi and blood. The qi cannot move through this yin dampness and it is said that blood and body fluids flow together. If one stops, so too tends the other.

28

Because damp depression may cause lack of free flow, dampness can also be a cause of pain.

If dampness gathers and lingers for a long time, or if it is worked on and transformed by either heat or cold, it may turn into phlegm. Phlegm is nothing other than congealed dampness. No matter what the cause of phlegm, once it is produced, it may hinder the free flow of the qi and blood. Thus it too may be associated with pain due to obstruction and impediment of free flow.

Not only is qi supposed to move and transform blood and body fluids, qi is also supposed to move and transform food. If the qi becomes depressed and stagnant, the digestate may not be moved. This yin substance then further blocks the free flow of qi and blood, and thus causes pain. This pain mostly occurs in the stomach and abdomen. So it is not a main cause of headache. However, if food becomes stagnant and accumulates for any reason, then this can aggravate any other cause or tendency to qi, blood, damp, or phlegm obstruction.

Qi is yang in nature and, therefore, is warm. If qi becomes depressed and accumulates, a lot of yang qi in one place may give rise to pathological heat. If there is enough heat, this is called evil fire. Fire's nature is to flare or flame upward. Therefore, depressive heat produced in the internal viscera, such as the liver, gallbladder, and stomach, often moves upward to accumulate in the head. If it becomes blocked there in the bony box of the skull, it will prevent the healthy or so-called righteous qi and blood from moving freely there. Thus there will be pain.

External causes

It is also possible for obstruction and blockage to be caused by what Chinese medicine calls external evils. If pathological qi (meaning influences) invade the body, they lodge in places they are not meant to be in. It is a basic axiom that two things cannot inhabit the same space. If one exists there, the other cannot. In

29

the same way, external evils which invade the body block and hinder the free flow of the righteous qi and blood. This results in pain.

Different natures, different types of pain

Depending on what is obstructed and what is doing the blocking, there are different types of pain. For instance, qi stagnation causes distended, bloated, full feelings of discomfort. Static blood is associated with fixed, localized pain which is sharp or piercing in nature or simply very severe in intensity. Dampness causes heavy, distended, tight, or full pain. Phlegm itself typically is painless. However, because it can block the free flow of qi and blood, phlegm obstruction may be associated with pain of either type. Pain associated with externally invading wind evils moves about, comes and goes, and mostly affects the upper body. It may also be associated with tingling, itching, or numbness. Pain associated with cold is typically fixed in location, intense, and chilly in nature. It also is benefitted by warmth. Pain associated with heat or fire is hot in nature and can also be quite intense. Besides heat, pain, and redness, there may also be swelling.

Pain which is due to something blocking and obstructing the free flow of qi and blood is called replete pain in Chinese medicine.

Insufficiency & weakness

Lack of free flow may also be due to either lack of qi to move blood and body fluids or lack of blood to fill the vessels. If qi vacuity and weakness is even more severe, it is called yang vacuity. Yang is merely a lot of qi in one place. If blood vacuity is more severe, it is called yin and/or essence insufficiency. Yin is nothing other than a lot of blood and essence in one place. Lack of free flow due to vacuity and insufficiency is called vacuity pain. Vacuity pain is typically not so severe. However, it tends to be enduring and persistent and is aggravated by exertion, fatigue, and loss of blood or body fluids.

Mixed repletion & vacuity

In real life, the body is very complex, and most people with disease present a mixture vacuity and repletion. For instance, if the spleen qi becomes vacuous and weak, then the qi may not move and transform body fluids. These then give rise to phlegm and dampness which obstruct and hinder the free flow of qi and blood. It is also possible for blood vacuity to give rise to blood stasis or blood stasis to give rise to blood vacuity. If there is insufficient blood to nourish and construct the vessels, the vessels may not do their duty of moving the blood. Thus static blood is engendered. Vice versa, another name for static blood is dry or dead blood. Static blood inhibits the engenderment and transformation of new or fresh blood. If blood vacuity lasts long enough, it will give rise to yin vacuity, since blood is part of yin fluids and essence. Therefore, it is easy to see that a given person's pain may be a mixture of vacuity and repletion causes and mechanisms.

How to stop pain in Chinese medicine

If all pain in the body can be reduced to lack of free flow, then all pain in the body can be treated by restoring the free flow. "If there is pain, there is no free flow. *If there is free flow, there is no pain.*" Therefore, the basic principle for stopping or alleviating pain in Chinese medicine is to promote the free flow. However, in order to do that, the practitioner must know whether that pain is due to obstruction and blockage or due to weakness and insufficiency. If it is due to blockage and obstruction, then one must open that obstruction and disinhibit that blockage. If the pain is due to weakness and insufficiency, one must further determine whether qi and yang are too weak to move the qi or whether blood and yin are so insufficient they cannot nourish and fill the vessels. In the former case one boosts the qi and invigorates yang. In the latter, one nourishes the blood, enriches yin, and fills the essence.

Having understood the basic mechanisms of pain according to Chinese medicine, now let us turn to the specific causes and mechanisms of pain in the head or headache.

The Causes & Mechanisms of Headache

We have seen above something about the Chinese medical conception of the cause and nature of pain. Now let's turn to the disease causes and mechanisms of headache specifically. Philippe Sionneau describes the basic mechanisms of headache in his book, *The Treatment of Disease in TCM, Vol. 1: Diseases of the Head and Face Including Mental/Emotional Disorders*, also published by Blue Poppy Press.[3]

1. Contraction of external evils

If one's defensive qi is weak but external evils are strong, these external evils may take advantage of this relative vacuity and weakness to enter and invade the body. The most common external evils to invade the body and cause headache are wind, cold, dampness, and heat. Typically in such cases, wind combines with either cold and dampness or with heat. In either case, these external evils lodge in the channels and network vessels of the head and face and inhibit the free flow of the qi and blood in the affected area. Since there is no free flow, there is pain.

2. Internal damage

The liver, spleen, and kidneys are the three viscera most commonly involved in this group of disease mechanisms leading to head pain.

---

[3] Sionneau, Philippe, *The Treatment of Disease in TCM, Vol. 1: Diseases of the Head and Face Including Mental/Emotional Disorders*, Blue Poppy Press, Boulder, CO, 1996

A. Every desire puts qi in motion. If a desire is unfulfilled, the qi it is an expression of is thwarted and is not able to flow to its hoped-for destination or conclusion. Since it is the liver which is responsible for maintaining the "coursing and discharging" of the qi, such unfulfilled desires can damage the liver and cause it not to function efficiently. In that case, the liver becomes "depressed" and the qi becomes stagnant. If the qi becomes stagnant, this means it backs up and accumulates. Since its nature is inherently yang, accumulated yang qi will tend to counterflow upward like steam escaping from a pressure cooker. When this upwardly counterflowing liver qi or liver yang arrives in the bony box of the head, it has no place to go and no easy way out. Because it takes the place of the qi and blood which normally flow through the channels and network vessels of the head, it inhibits the qi and blood within the head, and thus there is pain.

Stress is nothing other than wanting to do more than we have the time, energy, or wherewithal to accomplish. Therefore, stress is nothing other than a compromise of the free flow of our desires. We are trying to rush somewhere to be on time but we get stuck in traffic. We are trying to get out a report for our boss, but our computer breaks down. We want to go to the hockey game with friends, but we have to stay late at work. All stress is nothing other than competing desires, some of which we simply cannot fulfill. Therefore, the more stress, the more liver depression qi stagnation. Eventually, this accumulated yang qi has to go somewhere. If it goes upward, it commonly causes a headache.

B. According to Chinese medical theory, the brain is the "sea of marrow" which is nourished and enriched by blood and essence. Blood and essence are both relatively yin. If, due to aging, prolonged excessive activity and overtaxation, enduring disease, too much sex, or drug, alcohol, tobacco, or caffeine use, yin blood is consumed, yin may fail to nourish the network vessels of the brain. These network vessels will fail to do their job, which is to transport the qi and blood. Hence, the free flow of the qi and blood in the brain is inhibited and there is pain.

34

If, due to aging, enduring disease, excessive sex, or too many drugs, kidney yang becomes vacuous and insufficient, then there will not be enough yang qi to warm the body. Yang qi arises in the lower body and must ascend to the upper body to empower and warm the head. Cold is yin and constricting and congealing in nature. The qi and blood must be kept at a certain temperature for them to flow freely. If kidney yang is insufficient, therefore, the qi and blood flow in the brain may become inhibited or not freely flowing. Thus there is pain in the head.

C. The spleen can cause headaches of at least three different kinds. The function of the spleen can become damaged by overwork, too little exercise, too much thinking and especially worry, or by improper diet. In particular, the spleen is easily damaged by eating too many chilled, uncooked foods, too many damp foods, such as dairy products and oils and fats, and too much sugar. If the spleen becomes vacuous and weak, it may fail to move and transform body fluids. If these collect, they may transform into phlegm and dampness. If phlegm and dampness are wafted upward in the body, they may lodge in the channels and network vessels of the head, thus obstructing and hindering the free flow of qi and blood.

Secondly, the spleen is the source of qi and blood transformation and engenderment. This means that it is mainly the spleen which is in charge of digestion of food and the creation of qi and blood out of the refined essence of food and liquids. Therefore, if the spleen is vacuous, so also may be the qi. If the qi becomes vacuous and weak, it may not be sufficient to ascend upward to the head to move and push the blood and body fluids. Again there is no free flow, and again there is pain.

And lastly, if, for any reason, the spleen becomes vacuous and weak, it may not transform and engender sufficient blood. The blood is necessary to nourish the channels and vessels in the head. If these do not receive sufficient nourishment and enrichment, they may cease to function properly. Since their function is none other than to promote the flow of qi and blood, therefore, once again, there is no free flow, and consequently there is pain.

3. Blood stasis, roundworms & food retention

A. Static blood may result from local traumatic injury. Traumatic injury severs the channels and vessels. The blood then flows outside the vessels. Because the blood can only flow when it is inside the vessels, it becomes static. Static blood then obstructs the flow of fresh blood, qi, and body fluids. Hence there is pain. Static blood may also be caused by enduring disease affecting the free flow of the qi and body fluids. For instance, if there is stress causing liver depression qi stagnation, and the qi remains stagnant for a long time, eventually this will result in blood stasis as well. As it is said in Chinese, "If the qi moves, the blood moves. If the qi stops, the blood stops." Similarly, if body fluids accumulate for any reason, because they are yin substance, they will impede the free flow of yang qi. This means that eventually the qi will become stagnant and thereafter the blood as well.

B. Roundworms and food retention both may also be involved with headaches. Roundworms may obstruct the bile duct and impede the free flow of liver qi. In that case, roundworms cause or aggravate liver depression qi stagnation. If one overeats or eats very hard-to-digest foods, stagnant food may be retained in the stomach. This yin stagnant food impedes the uninhibited, free flow of the qi. This then damages the liver and gives rise to or worsens qi stagnation. If this accumulated, stagnant qi ascends and counterflows to the head, then the free flow of the qi and blood in the head will be compromised. No free flow equals pain.

According to Chinese medical theory, no headache falls outside one of these causes and mechanisms. Commonly, headaches may be a combination of more than one of these mechanisms. For instance, stress may cause a predisposition to liver depression qi stagnation and yang qi may be tending to vent itself upward.

36

Therefore, there may be chronically tight shoulders and neck and a tendency to headache. If one then catches a cold, *i.e.*, a wind cold external invasion, this may constrict and congeal the qi and blood in the head enough to now trigger a headache. Likewise, it is very common for liver depression due to stress to be complicated by blood vacuity due to a weak spleen in turn due to loss of blood associated with menstruation, overwork, and a faulty diet. Another possibility is for liver depression qi stagnation to become complicated by phlegm dampness due to poor spleen function again due to faulty diet and/or too little exercise.

Enlightenment & empowerment

The beauty of this theory is that is does identify in very real terms what are the mechanisms of any individual's headache. If one knows that their headache is caused by phlegm dampness blocking the channels and networks vessels in the head, then there are steps one can take to transform this phlegm and eliminate this dampness. More importantly, there are also steps one can take in order to prevent the creation of such phlegm and dampness in the future. Therefore, Chinese medicine is both enlightening—it tells you why you are getting the kind of headaches you are—and it is empowering. Based on this identification of the causes of your particular headaches, there are real life steps you can take to stop them when you have them *and* prevent them from occurring again.

6

The Chinese Medical Treatment of Headache

The hallmark of professional Chinese medicine is what is known as "treatment based on pattern discrimination." Modern Western medicine bases its treatment on a disease diagnosis. This means that two patients diagnosed as suffering from the same disease will get the same treatment. Traditional Chinese medicine also takes the patient's disease diagnosis into account. However, the choice of treatment is not based on the disease so much as it is on what is called the patient's pattern, and it is treatment based on pattern discrimination which is what makes Chinese medicine the holistic, safe, and effective medicine it is.

In order to explain the difference between a disease and pattern, let us take headache for example. Everyone who is diagnosed as suffering from a headache has to, by definition, have some pain in their head. In modern Western medicine and other medical systems which primarily prescribe on the basis of a disease diagnosis, one can talk about "headache medicines." However, amongst headache sufferers, one may be a man and the other a woman. One may be old and the other young. One may be fat and the other skinny. One may have pain on the right side of her head and the other may have pain on the left. In one case, the pain may be throbbing and continuous, while the other person's pain may be very sharp but intermittent. In one case, they may also have indigestion, a tendency to loose stools, lack of warmth in their feet, red eyes, a dry mouth and desire for cold drinks, while the other person has a wet, weeping, crusty skin rash with red borders, a tendency to hay fever, ringing in their ears, and dizziness when they stand up. In Chinese medicine just as in modern Western medicine, both these patients suffer from headache. That is their disease diagnosis. However, they also suffer from a whole host of other complaints, have very different types of headaches, and very different constitutions, ages, and sex. In Chinese medicine, the patient's pattern is made up from all these other signs and symptoms and other information. Thus, in Chinese medicine, the pattern describes *the totality of the person as a unique individual*. And in Chinese medicine, treatment is designed to rebalance that entire pattern of imbalance as well as address the major complaint or disease. Thus, there is a saying in Chinese medicine:

> One disease, different treatments
> Different diseases, same treatment

This means that, in Chinese medicine, two patients with the same named disease diagnosis may receive different treatments *if their Chinese medical patterns are different*, while two patients diagnosed with different named diseases may receive the same treatment *if their Chinese medical pattern is the same*. In other words, in Chinese medicine, treatment is predicated primarily on one's pattern discrimination, not on one's named disease diagnosis. Therefore, each person is treated individually.

Since every patient gets just the treatment which is right to restore balance to their particular body, there are also no unwanted side effects. Side effects come from forcing one part of the body to behave while causing an imbalance in some other part. The medicine may have fit part of the problem but not the entirety of the patient as an individual. This is like robbing Peter to pay Paul. Since Chinese medicine sees the entire body (and mind!) as a single, unified whole, curing imbalance in one area of the body while causing it in another is unacceptable.

The following pattern discrimination for headaches also comes from Philippe Sionneau's *The Treatment of Disease in TCM, Vol. 1.*

The TCM pattern discrimination of headaches

1. Wind cold

Symptoms: Recurrent attacks that refer to the back of the neck and upper back, a feeling as if the back were girdled, aversion to wind, fear of cold, exacerbation by exposure to cold, no thirst, thin, white tongue fur, and a floating, tight pulse. This kind of headache typically occurs with a common cold, with airborne allergy attacks, and the beginnings of sinusitis.

Therapeutic principles: Resolve the exterior, dispel wind, and scatter cold

2. Wind heat

Symptoms: Headache accompanied by distention or even a splitting sensation, fever, aversion to wind, flushed red facial complexion, red eyes, thirst with desire to drink, constipation, dark colored urine, a red tongue with yellow fur, and a floating, rapid pulse. This kind of headache goes along with common colds and the beginnings of sinusitis.

Therapeutic principles: Course wind and clear heat, open the network vessels and stop pain

3. Wind dampness

Symptoms: Headache characterized as the sensation of something tight bound around the head, dizziness and heaviness of the head, worse in damp, wet weather, chest oppression, epigastric fullness, poor appetite, heavy limbs with lack of strength, scanty urination, loose stools, slimy, white tongue fur, and a soggy, slippery pulse

Therapeutic principles: Dispel wind and overcome dampness, open the network vessels and stop pain

4. Ascendant liver yang hyperactivity

Symptoms: Headache with dizziness or vertigo, headache commonly located in the temporal regions or top of the head, vexation and agitation, irritability, restless sleep, possible lateral costal pain, tinnitus, a flushed red face, a bitter taste in the mouth, a red tongue with scanty or scanty, yellow fur, and a wiry, forceful pulse. This pattern of headache may be found in migraine sufferers and people with hypertension. It may also be found in those with chronic, recurrent tension headaches.

Therapeutic principles: Level the liver, subdue yang, and stop pain

5. Exuberant liver fire

Symptoms: Headache with a distended feeling in the head, headache often located at the top of the head, irritability, tinnitus, occasional pain and a sensation of heat in the lateral costal region, red eyes, dryness and a bitter taste in the mouth, dark colored urine, constipation, yellow tongue fur, and a wiry, rapid pulse. This pattern may be seen in those with migraines, hypertension, sinusitis, and trigeminal neuralgia.

Therapeutic principles: Clear the liver, drain fire, and stop pain

6. Kidney yin vacuity

Symptoms: Headache characterized by an empty sensation in the head, vexatious heat, dry throat, dizziness, low back and knee soreness and weakness, lassitude of the spirit, seminal emission, loss of sleep, a red tongue with scant fur, and a fine, forceless pulse

Therapeutic principles: Enrich yin and supplement the kidneys, stop pain

7. Kidney yang vacuity

Symptoms: A dull headache and sometimes a cold sensation in the head, pain worsened by cold, fear of cold, chilled limbs, a pale white facial complexion, a pale tongue, and a deep and fine or deep and slow pulse

Therapeutic principles: Warm and supplement kidney yang, stop pain

8. Blood vacuity

Symptoms: Dull headache with dizziness, heart palpitations, rubbing of the eyes and blurred vision, insomnia or scanty sleep, lassitude of the spirit, a pale white facial complexion, pale lips, pale nails, a pale tongue, and a fine, weak pulse. Often, blood vacuity headaches occur after menstruation or when very fatigued or they may be complicated by liver yang hyperactivity.

Therapeutic principles: Nourish the blood and harmonize the network vessels, stop pain

9. Qi vacuity

Symptoms: Dull headache with an empty sensation in the head which is worsened by overtaxation, sweating on exertion, lassitude of the spirit, susceptibility to the contraction of external evils, poor appetite, shortness of breath, loose stools, scanty, white tongue fur, and a vacuous, forceless pulse. This pattern of headache occurs when the person is fatigued or has overworked.

Therapeutic principles: Supplement the center and boost the qi, stop pain

10. Damp phlegm

Symptoms: Headache with dizziness, epigastric fullness, chest oppression, a possible heavy sensation in the body, vomiting of phlegm drool, poor appetite, lassitude of the spirit, slimy, white tongue fur, and a wiry, slippery pulse

43

Therapeutic principles: Fortify the spleen and transform phlegm, open the network vessels and stop pain

11. Blood stasis

Symptoms: Obstinate, pricking headache with fixed location, a history of trauma or as a result of enduring disease, a purple tongue with scant, white fur, and a fine and choppy, or deep and choppy pulse. Blood stasis may complicate a number of these other patterns. This is because blood stasis tends to occur whenever there is enduring or long-lasting disease. Therefore, if one has had chronic, recurrent headaches for a long time, they should look for signs and symptoms of blood stasis along with the symptoms of other patterns.

Therapeutic principles: Quicken the blood and transform stasis, move the qi and stop pain

12. Roundworms

Symptoms: Headache, vexation and oppression, vomiting, paroxysmal abdominal pain, possible vomiting of roundworms, worm macules on the face, miliary dots on the inner surface of the lips, and a wiry, slippery pulse. Although roundworm infestation is a possible cause of headache, it is not, in my experience a commonly found pattern amongst North American patients.

Therapeutic principles: Quiet the roundworms and stop pain

13. Food retention

Symptoms: Headache, fullness in the chest and epigastrium, aversion to food, acid regurgitation, belching of putrid gas, thick, slimy tongue fur, and a wiry pulse. Food retention headaches are usually associated with a particular episode of eating and drinking too much. Food stagnation is not usually associated with chronic, recurrent headaches.

Therapeutic principles: Disperse food and abduct stagnation

You can see from the above pattern descriptions with their treatment principles, each different pattern of headache sufferer requires different treatment principles to bring them back into balance. In other words, there is no single headache remedy in Chinese medicine, and a remedy which is just right for one pattern might actually make the sufferer with another pattern worse.

Most chronic, recurrent headaches are associated with liver yang hyperactivity, kidney yin vacuity, blood vacuity, qi vacuity, and phlegm dampness. Likewise, in clinical practice, most patients with chronic, recurrent headaches have a combination of more than one pattern. For instance, in women with menstrual migraine headaches, it is not uncommon to find liver yang hyperactivity with blood vacuity and blood stasis. Another common menstrual migraine pattern is qi and blood vacuity with blood stasis. In heavy-set, overweight men and women, it is not uncommon to find a combination of liver yang hyperactivity with phlegm and dampness. Therefore, in real life, the above simple TCM patterns do have to be modified to fit individual patients individually.

How This System Works in Real Life

Using all the above information on the theory of Chinese medicine and the patterns and their mechanisms of headache let's see how a Chinese doctor makes this system work in real life.

Take Jean, for example, who we introduced at the beginning of this book. She has experienced migraine headaches on and off since she was about 13. Typically Jean's migraines occur at the onset of her menstrual periods. They can also occur any time she is under a lot of stress or if she eats peanuts and chocolate. Her migraines are preceded by a visual aura and tingling and numbness on her face and hands. The pain is pounding and located always on the left side. During an attack, she cannot stand any light or sound. At some point in a migrainous attack, Jean gets so nauseous she vomits and often also experiences diarrhea. After she vomits and/or has diarrhea, she can usually fall asleep. When Jean wakes up, the headache is gone. In terms of menstruation, Jean reports that she does have PMS. She gets irritable and is easily angered for a week before each menses. In addition, her breasts get swollen and sore and her nipples get especially sensitive during that same time.

When I ask to see Jean's tongue, it appears puffy. It is generally a bit paler than normal, but the tip and left edge are redder than normal. Jean's pulse is bowstring, fine, and a bit rapid. It also feels soggy over her wrist bone on the right side. Bowstring and soggy are two of the 28 standard pulse images or descriptions of

Chinese medicine. A bowstring pulse feels like a taut wire, while a soggy pulse is floating, fine, and forceless.

How a Chinese doctor analyzes Jean's symptoms

Jean's premenstrual irritability, her swollen, sore breasts, and her hypersensitive nipples all point towards liver depression qi stagnation. This is corroborated by her bowstring pulse. However, in Jean's case, there is also blood vacuity. We know this because her tongue is generally paler than normal and her pulse is also fine. This blood vacuity is due to spleen weakness. We know this because of the slightly puffy tongue and the soggy pulse over the right wrist bone, the pulse position corresponding to the spleen. Jean's liver depression qi stagnation gets worse in the week before her menses arrive because the body's blood collects in the uterus for expulsion with the period. If the blood is vacuous and insufficient, this does not leave enough left over to perform its proper functions in the rest of the body. Since the liver can only function if it receives blood to nourish it, the liver's coursing and discharging becomes even more dysfunctional during the premenstruum. This is why Jean gets PMS and why her migraines are mostly associated with her periods. The fact that she gets her migraines on the left side also confirms this. The left side corresponds to the blood.

Because Jean's liver depression qi stagnation gets worse before her menses, the stagnant qi tends to transform into heat or hyperactive yang. This is confirmed by the rapid pulse and the red tongue tip and left side pain, the left side also corresponding to the liver. This accumulated liver qi which has transformed into hyperactive liver yang has to go somewhere. So it counterflows upward along the yang channel connected to the liver, the gallbladder and triple burner channels. These two channels traverse the sides of the head.

Some of the liver qi also vents horizontally to attack the stomach and spleen. When the liver attacks the stomach, there is nausea and even vomiting. If the liver qi attacks the spleen, there may be diarrhea. If there is vomiting or diarrhea, however, a lot of qi is bled off or discharged with the vomitus and stools. This is like releasing the safety valve on a pressure cooker. The liver qi is vented outside the body and, therefore, it does not need to counterflow upward into the bony box of the head. Hence, the headache subsides. Because Jean has vented a lot of qi, she also falls asleep.

The tingling around the mouth and hands show that A) there is blood vacuity, and B) that the qi is starting to move in the body chaotically like wind rushing here and there. The visual aura and photophobia both have to do with the liver. The eyes are the portals of the liver. The eyes can see only when they receive sufficient blood to nourish them. The flashing lights, dazzling lines, etc., that many migraineurs "see" are manifestations of the yang qi flooding the head from the liver. The fact that the patient cannot stand any outside light or noise has to do with both of these stimuli being species of yang qi entering the head from outside. There is already way too much yang qi pounding inside Jean's head to tolerate any more entering from outside.

The fact that nuts and chocolate can both sometimes trigger a migraine attack is due to their being oily, fatty foods. Oil and fat are damp and hot. Hyperactivity of liver yang is also hot. Heat added to heat makes that heat worse. In addition, cocoa is considered hot and particularly inflames that heat in the body which is the "pilot light" for liver yang.

If we put this all together, the Chinese doctor knows that there is liver depression transforming into liver yang hyperactivity which then counterflows upward into the head. This liver depression is aggravated by blood vacuity, and this blood vacuity is aggravated by the menstrual cycle since the blood is sent downward to the uterus from the premenstruum through the period itself.

How a Chinese doctor treats Jean's headache

Jean's case is characterized by two phases. There is the time between migraine attacks when Jean is "normal" and there are the attacks themselves. Between attacks, the Chinese doctor will attempt to course Jean's liver and rectify her qi, supplement her spleen and nourish her blood. Since the liver yang hyperactivity causing the migraines transforms from liver depression qi stagnation and is aggravated by blood vacuity in turn due to spleen vacuity, these principles are formulated to try to prevent further occurrences of Jean's migraines by treating the root mechanisms of her head pain.

During the attacks themselves, the treatment principles are to clear liver heat, downbear upward counterflow, subdue yang, and nourish the blood. In other words, Jean's Chinese medical treatment is also divided into two phases. Phase one attempts to treat the underlying root mechanisms of Jean's migraines during the time she otherwise seems normal. Phase two occurs during the premenstruum and the menses themselves and attempts to stop or prevent the migraines during the time they are most likely to occur.

Once the Chinese doctor has stated the treatment principles necessary for re-establishing balance within the organism, then they know that anything which works to accomplish these principles will be good for the patient. Using these principles, the Chinese doctor can now select various acupuncture points which achieve these effects. They can prescribe Chinese herbal medicinals which embody these principles. They can make recommendations about what to eat and not eat based on these principles. They can make recommendations on lifestyle changes. And, in short, they can advise the patient on *any and every aspect of their life*, judging whether something either aids the accomplishment of these principles or works against it.

In Chinese medicine, the internal administration of Chinese "herbal" medicinals is the main modality.[4] So let's look at how a Chinese doctor crafts a prescription for Jean. Because the first treatment principles stated for Jean were to course the liver and rectify the qi, supplement the spleen and nourish the blood, the Chinese doctor knows that he or she should select their guiding formula from the harmonizing the liver and spleen category of formulas. Depending on the textbook, there are 22-28 main categories of formulas in Chinese medicine, each category correlated to a main treatment principle. The category of harmonizing the liver and spleen, is part of a broader category of harmonizing formulas which are used to treat patterns that involve complex processes in different levels of the body, different organs, as well as the presence of hot and cold simultaneously.

Under this category of formulas, there is one very famous formula which addresses all of the above treatment principles we have said are necessary, *Xiao Yao San* (Rambling Powder). This formula can be used for a wide variety of complaints characterized, on the one hand, by liver depression qi stagnation, and, on the other hand, spleen vacuity giving rise to blood vacuity. The Chinese doctor would then modify this prescription to address the specific patient's complaints more effectively.

The standard formula is comprised of:

Radix Bupleri (*Chai Hu*)
Radix Albus Paeoniae Lactiflorae (*Bai Shao*)
Radix Angelicae Sinensis (*Dang Gui*)
Rhizoma Atractylodis Macrocephalae (*Bai Zhu*)
Sclerotium Poriae Cocos (*Fu Ling*)

---

[4] We've put the word herbal in quotation marks since Chinese medicine is not entirely herbal. Herbs are medicinals made from parts of plants, their roots, bark, stems, leaves, flowers, etc. Chinese medicinals are mostly herbal in nature. However, a percentage of Chinese medicinals also come from the animal and mineral realms. Thus not all Chinese medicinals are, strictly speaking, herbs.

Herba Menthae Haplocalycis (*Bo He*)
mix-fried Radix Glycyrrhizae *(Gan Cao)*
uncooked Rhizoma Zingiberis *(Sheng Jiang)*

Bupleurum courses the liver, rectifies the qi, and resolves depression. White Peony and Dang Gui both nourish the blood. By nourishing the blood, they also soften and harmonize the liver. Atractylodes and Poria supplement the spleen so it can transform and engender the blood. In addition, Poria leads any yang qi or evil heat downward in the body rather than up. Mentha helps Bupleurum course the liver and resolve depression. Both are somewhat cooling. So they keep liver depression from transforming into depressive heat or hyperactive yang. Uncooked Ginger assists Bupleurum in moving the qi, while it assists Atractylodes and Poria is getting rid of any dampness that may hinder the functioning of the spleen. And finally, Glycyrrhiza or Licorice supplements the spleen, nourishes heart blood, and calms the spirit, while also harmonizing all the other ingredients into a cohesive, healthful whole.

This formula might be given to Jean from the time of ovulation onward till day 21 or the onset of any premenstrual symptoms. Usually, a formula such as this would be taken two to three times each day. The herbs would be soaked in water and then boiled into a very strong "tea" for 30-45 minutes.

During the premenstruum itself, the Chinese doctor would probably switch Jean to a different formula, one which is specifically for liver yang hyperactivity. One such formula is *Tian Ma Gou Teng Yin* (Gastrodia & Uncaria Drink). It's ingredients include:

Rhizoma Gastrodiae Elatae *(Tian Ma)*
Ramulus Uncariae Cum Uncis *(Gou Teng)*
Concha Haliotidis *(Shi Jue Ming)*
Ramulus Loranthi Seu Visci *(Sang Ji Sheng)*
Cortex Eucommiae Ulmoidis *(Du Zhong)*

Radix Cyathulae (*Chuan Niu Xi*)
Fructus Gardeniae Jasminoidis (*Shan Zhi Zi*)
Radix Scutellariae Baicalensis (*Huang Qin*)
Herba Leonuri Heterophylli (*Yi Mu Cao*)
Caulis Polygoni Multiflori (*Ye Jiao Teng*)
Sclerotium Poriae Cocos (*Fu Ling*)

Within this formula, Gastrodia and Uncaria both level liver wind, while Uncaria clears liver heat. Liver wind means chaotically counterflowing liver qi ascending to the head and running around in the skin. Loranthus and Eucommia both nourish the blood and supplement the kidneys. The kidneys are the mother of the liver and the blood is the mother of qi. Supplementing the blood and kidneys helps to control liver yang. Cyathula leads the qi to move downward, not up. So does Poria. Gardenia and Scutellaria both clear heat from the liver. Leonurus quickens the blood and transforms stasis. If there is long-term liver depression qi stagnation, there is often at least an element of blood stasis. And Caulis Polygoni Multiflori courses the liver and resolves depression, nourishes the heart and quiets the spirit. Because the headache occurs on the side of the head and in order to make this formula even more powerful in moving the qi and blood in the head, one might add some Radix Ligustici Wallichii (*Chuan Xiong*) to the above prescription.

The ingredients in these two formulas may also be taken as a dried, powdered extract. Such extracts are manufactured by several Taiwanese and Japanese companies. Although such extracts are not, in my experience, as powerful as the freshly decocted "teas", they are easier to take. Many standard formulas also come as ready-made pills. However, these cannot be modified. If their ingredients match the individual patient's requirements, then they are fine. If the formula needs modifications, then teas or powders whose individual ingredients can be added and subtracted are necessary.

In exactly the same way, the practitioner of Chinese medicine could create an individualized acupuncture treatment plan and would certainly create an accompanying dietary and lifestyle plan. However, we will discuss each of these in their own chapter.

In a woman with Jean's Chinese pattern discrimination and long history of migraines, we can expect that she will need to take the Chinese herbal medicine for at least three months or menstrual cycles. After that, she may want to go back on one or the other of these formulas whenever she is under special stress. However, the main preventive treatment is identifying the dietary and lifestyle factors which get her into trouble in the first place and then modifying or avoiding these. Migraines are not something that can be cured once like measles and then you are home free the rest of your life. Jean will still have to be careful until she passes through menopause at least. However, she should now know much better what she can do for herself, and she also will know that there is Chinese medicine which can help her when times get rough and stress is unavoidable.

Chinese Herbal Medicine & Headaches

As we have seen from Jean's case above, there is no Chinese "anti-headache herb" or even a single "anti-headache formula" which will work for all sufferers of depression. Chinese medicinals are individually prescribed based on a person's pattern discrimination, not on a disease diagnosis like headache. Patients often come to practitioners of Chinese medicine saying, "My friend told me that *Xiao Yao Wan* (Rambling Pills, a common Chinese over the counter medication) is good for PMS. But I tried it and it didn't work." This is because *Xiao Yao Wan* is meant to treat a *specific pattern* of PMS, not PMS per se. If you exhibit that pattern, then this formula will work. If you do not have signs and symptoms of this pattern, it won't.

In addition, because most people's headaches are a combination of different Chinese patterns and disease mechanisms, professional Chinese medicine never treats headaches with herbal "singles." In herbalism, singles mean the prescription of a single herb all by itself. Chinese herbal medicine is based on rebalancing patterns, and patterns in real life patients almost always have more than a single element. Therefore, Chinese doctors almost always prescribe herbs in multi-ingredient formulas. Such formulas may have anywhere from six to 18 or more ingredients. When a practitioner of Chinese medicine reads a prescription by another practitioner, they can tell you not only what the patient's pattern discrimination is but also their probable signs and symptoms. In other words, the practitioner of Chinese medicine does not just combine several medicinals which are all reputed to be "good for headache." Rather, they carefully craft a formula whose ingredients are meant to rebalance every aspect of the patient's bodymind.

Getting your own individualized prescription

Since, in China, it takes not less than four years of full-time college education to learn how to do a professional Chinese pattern discrimination and then write an herbal formula based on that pattern discrimination, most laypeople cannot realistically write their own Chinese herbal prescriptions. It should also be remembered that Chinese herbs are not effective and safe because they are either Chinese or herbal. In fact, approximately 20% of the common Chinese materia medica did not originate in China, and not all Chinese herbs are completely safe. They are only safe when prescribed according to a correct pattern discrimination, in the right dose, and for the right amount of time. After all, if an herb is strong enough to heal and imbalance, it is also strong enough to create an imbalance if overdosed or misprescribed. Therefore, I strongly recommend persons who wish to experience the many benefits of Chinese herbal medicine to see a qualified professional practitioner who can do a professional pattern discrimination and write you an individualized prescription. Towards the end of this book, I give the reader suggestions on how to find a qualified professional Chinese medical practitioner near you.

Experimenting with Chinese patent medicines

In reality, qualified professional practitioners of Chinese medicine are not yet found in every North American community. In addition, some people may want to try to heal their headaches as much on their own as possible. More and more health food stores are stocking a variety of ready-made Chinese formulas in pill and powder form. These ready-made, over-the-counter Chinese medicines are often referred to as Chinese patent medicines. Although my best recommendation is for readers to seek Chinese herbal treatment from professional practitioners, below are some suggestions of how one might experiment with Chinese patent medicines to treat headache.

In chapter 6, I have given the signs and symptoms of the 13 basic patterns associated with most people's headache. These are:

1. Wind cold
2. Wind heat
3. Wind dampness
4. Hyperactivity of ascendant liver yang
5. Exuberant liver fire
6. Kidney yin vacuity
7. Kidney yang vacuity
8. Blood vacuity
9. Qi vacuity
10. Damp phlegm
11. Blood stasis
12. Roundworms
13. Food retention

If the reader can identify their main pattern from chapter 6, then there are some Chinese patent remedies that they might consider trying.

Chuan Xiong Cha Tiao Wan

This Chinese patent medicine deserves to be kept in every family's medicine closet. Its name translates as Ligusticum & Tea Mixed Pills. It is a specific remedy for wind cold headache. However, because it contains a number of ingredients which move the qi and quicken the blood in the various channels which traverse the head and face, it can be used for first-aid purposes for most replete kinds of head and face pain. For instance, this formula also treats wind damp headache. Its ingredients include:

Radix Ligustici Wallichii (*Chuan Xiong*)
Radix Et Rhizoma Notopterygii (*Qiang Huo*)
Radix Angelicae Dahuricae (*Bai Zhi*)
Herba Asari Cum Radice (*Xi Xin*)
Herba Seu Flos Schizonepetae Tenuifoliae (*Jing Jie Sui*)
Radix Ledebouriellae Divaricatae (*Fang Feng*)
Herba Menthae Haplocalycis (*Bo He*)

Radix Glycyrrhizae (*Gan Cao*)
Folium Camilliae Chinensis (*Cha Ye*)

Notopterygium, Angelica, Schizonepeta, Ledebouriella, Mentha, and Camilliae (*i.e.*, tea leaves) all resolve the exterior and scatter wind. The first four of these are warm in nature and also scatter cold. The last two are cool in nature and clear heat. Asarum is quite warm and enters the tiniest network vessels in order to quicken the blood. Ligusticum also quickens the blood and especially in the head. Glycyrrhiza or Licorice harmonizes all the ingredients in the formula and helps them not create any side effects and especially digestive side effects.

These pills can be taken along with other Chinese patent medicines corresponding to other patterns in order to help them more effectively treat the symptoms of pain in the head. These pills should not, however, be used with yin or blood vacuity, since the ingredients in this formula are very drying and tend to consume and damage blood and yin in those with a yin vacuous bodily constitution.

Sang Ju Yin

This formula, called Morus & Chrysanthemum Drink in English, is the standard guiding formula for wind heat common cold and cough where there is also an element of dryness. However, it does also include at least two ingredients for treating hot-natured headaches. Its ingredients include:

Folium Mori Albi (*Sang Ye*)
Flos Chyrsanthemi Morifolii (*Ju Hua*)
Herba Menthae Haplocalycis (*Bo He*)
Semen Pruni Armeniacae (*Xing Ren*)
Radix Platycodi Grandiflori (*Jie Geng*)
Fructus Forsythiae Suspensae (*Lian Qiao*)
Rhizoma Phragmitis Communis (*Lu Gen*)
Radix Glycyrrhizae (*Gan Cao*)

Morus and Chrysanthemum both clear heat from the head, face, and eyes. They resolve the exterior and effuse wind while also clearing heat. Externally invading wind heat often stirs up or compounds any existing liver heat. Both these two medicinals not only address wind heat but also liver heat and yang hyperactivity. They are assisted by Mentha which also resolves the exterior and clears heat, whether exterior heat or liver heat. Armeniaca transforms phlegm, moistens dryness, and stops coughing. Playtcodon also transforms phlegm and stops coughing. Forsythia resolves the exterior and clears heat. Phragmites engenders stomach and intestinal fluids. And Licorice harmonizes the entire formula while also clearing some heat on its own. Because Armeniaca and Phragmites both enrich the stomach and engender fluids in the bowels, they promote the free flow of the stools. Constipation is very likely in this pattern. If the bowels move downward, then this relieves pressure and pain in the head. In this case, taking an enema can also help relieve the headache as well as the other symptoms of this pattern.

Xin Yi Wan

Called Magnolia Flower Pills in English, these pills are especially effective for relieving blocked nasal passages and sinus pressure due to wind damp invasion. Their ingredients are:

Flos Magnoliae Lilleflorae (*Xin Yi*)
Rhizoma Atractylodis Macrocephalae (*Bai Zhu*)
Radix Ledebouriellae Divaricatae (*Fang Feng*)
Herba Asari Cum Radice (*Xi Xin*)
Radix Et Rhizoma Notopterygii (*Qiang Huo*)
Radix Et Rhizoma Ligustici Sinensis (*Gao Ben*)
Radix Ligustici Wallichii (*Chuan Xiong*)
Rhizoma Cimicifugae (*Sheng Ma*)
Caulis Akebiae (*Mu Tong*)
Radix Glycyrrhizae (*Gan Cao*)

Bi Yan Pian

These pills' name means Rhinitis Tablets in English. They are for acute or chronic rhinitis, sinusitis with runny nose and large amounts of thick, yellow, pussy discharge, stuffy nose, hay fever, and the headache that accompanies such symptoms. In terms of Chinese pattern discrimination, these tablets treat wind heat.[5] Their ingredients are:

Fructus Xanthii Sibirici (*Cang Er Zi*)
Flos Magnoliae Lilleflorae (*Xin Yi*)
Radix Glycyrrhizae (*Gan Cao*)
Cortex Phellodendri (*Huang Bai*)
Radix Platycodi Grandiflori (*Jie Geng*)
Fructus Schisandrae Chinensis (*Wu Wei Zi*)
Fructus Forsythiae Suspensae (*Lian Qiao*)
Radix Angelicae Dahuricae (*Bai Zhi*)
Rhizoma Anemarrhenae Aspheloidis (*Zhi Mu*)
Flos Chrysanthemi Indici (*Ye Ju Hua*)
Radix Ledebouriellae Divaricatae (*Fang Feng*)
Herba Seu Flos Schizonepetae Tenuifoliae (*Jing Jie Sui*)

Do not exceed the recommended dosage of these pills as stated on the packaging.

Huo Xiang Zheng Qi Wan

These pills' name translates as Agastaches Correct the Qi Pills. They are based on a very old and very famous formula for summerheat flu. This means that they treat wind damp heat. The symptoms of this are fever, chills, headache, upper abdominal distention, abdominal pain, nausea, vomiting, flatulence, and either diarrhea or sticky, incomplete stools. The tongue fur is white and slimy. The ingredients in this formula include:

---

[5] The Chung Lian brand of this formula contains acetaminophen.

Herba Agastachis Seu Pogostemi (*Huo Xiang*)
Radix Angelicae Dahuricae (*Bai Zhi*)
Pericarpium Arecae Catechu (*Da Fu Pi*)
Folium Perillae Frutescentis (*Zi Su Ye*)
Sclerotium Poriae Cocos (*Fu Ling*)
Rhizoma Atractylodis Macrocephalae (*Bai Zhu*)
Cortex Magnoliae Officinalis (*Hou Po*)
Radix Platycodi Grandiflori (*Jie Geng*)
Pericarpium Citri Reticulatae (*Chen Pi*)
Radix Glycyrrhizae (*Gan Cao*)

Xiao Yao Wan (also spelled *Hsiao Yao Wan*)

Xiao Yao Wan is one of the most common Chinese herbal formulas prescribed. Its Chinese name has been translated as Free & Easy Pills, Rambling Pills, Relaxed Wanderer Pills, and several other versions of this same idea of promoting a freer and smoother, more relaxed flow. As a patent medicine, this formula comes as pills, and there are both Chinese-made and American-made versions of this formula available over the counter in the North American marketplace.[6]

The ingredients in this formula are:

Radix Bupleuri (*Chai Hu*)
Radix Angelicae Sinensis (*Dang Gui*)
Radix Albus Paeoniae Lactiflorae (*Bai Shao*)
Rhizoma Atractylodis Macrocephalae (*Bai Zhu*)
Sclerotium Poriae Cocos (*Fu Ling*)
mix-fried Radix Glycyrrhizae (*Gan Cao*)
Herba Menthae Haplocalycis (*Bo He*)
uncooked Rhizoma Zingiberis (*Sheng Jiang*)

---

[6] When marketed as a dried, powdered extract, this formula is sold under the name of Bupleurum & Tang-kuei Formula.

This formula treats the pattern of liver depression qi stagnation complicated by blood vacuity and spleen weakness with possible dampness as well. Bupleurum courses the liver and rectifies the qi. It is aided in this by Mentha. Dang Gui and White Peony nourish the blood and soften and harmonize the liver. Atractylodes and Poria fortify the spleen and eliminate dampness. Mix-fried Licorice aids these two in fortifying the spleen and supplementing the liver, while uncooked Ginger aids in both promoting and regulating the qi flow and eliminating dampness.

Liver depression qi stagnation per se is not one of the patterns of headache described by Philippe Sionneau above. However, this pattern typically precedes liver yang hyperactivity. Therefore, this formula can be taken in order to undercut the tendency for liver depression to transform into liver heat or hyperactivity. The symptoms of this pattern include chest and rib-side distention and pain, irritability, chest oppression, emotional depression, a tendency to sigh, premenstrual breast distention and soreness, possible premenstrual lower abdominal distention and cramping, a normal or slightly dark tongue with a thin, white coating, and a bowstring pulse.[7]

Because Bupleurum is very drying and also upbearing, after taking these pills at the dose recommended on the packaging, if one notices any side effects, then stop immediately and seek a professional consultation. Such side effects from this formula might include nervousness, irritability, a dry mouth and increased thirst, provocation or worsening of headaches, and red, dry eyes. Such side effects show that this formula, at least without modification, is not right for you. Although it may be doing you some good, it is also causing some harm. Remember, Chinese medicine is meant to cure without side effects, and as

---

[7] Feng Cun-wei in a recent article in *Xin Zhong Yi (New Chinese Medicine)* on neurovascular headaches actually does list liver qi depression and binding as a pattern of such headaches.

long as the prescription matches one's pattern there will not be any.

Dan Zhi Xiao Yao Wan

Dan Zhi Xiao Yao Wan or Moutan & Gardenia Rambling Pills is a modification of the above formula which also comes as a patent medicine in the form of pills.[8] It is meant to treat the pattern of liver depression transforming into heat with spleen vacuity and possible blood vacuity and/or dampness. The ingredients in this formula are the same as above except that two other herbs are added:

Cortex Radicis Moutan (*Dan Pi*)
Fructus Gardeniae Jasminoidis (*Shan Zhi Zi*)

These two ingredients clear heat and resolve depression. In addition, Moutan quickens the blood and dispels stasis and is good at clearing heat specifically from the blood.

Basically, the signs and symptoms of the pattern for which this formula is designed are the same as those for *Xiao Yao Wan* above plus signs and symptoms of depressive heat. These might include a reddish tongue with slightly yellow fur, a bowstring and rapid pulse, a bitter taste in the mouth, and increased irritability. It is my experience that this pattern may present especially in women with menstrual migraines or one-sided headaches.

Tian Ma Gou Teng Wan

The name of these pills translates as Gastrodia & Uncaria Pills. They are the standard textbook formula for ascendant hyperactivity of liver yang. Their ingredients include:

---

[8] When marketed as a dried, powdered extract, this formula is called Bupleurum & Peony Formula.

Rhizoma Gastrodiae Elatae (*Tian Ma*)
Ramulus Uncariae Cum Uncis (*Gou Teng*)
Concha Haliotidis (*Shi Jue Ming*)
Ramulus Loranthi Seu Visci (*Sang Ji Sheng*)
Cortex Eucommiae Ulmoidis (*Du Zhong*)
Fructus Gardeniae Jasminoidis (*Shan Zhi Zi*)
Radix Scutellariae Baicalensis (*Huang Qin*)
Radix Cyathulae (*Chuan Niu Xi*)
Herba Leonuri Heterophylli (*Yi Mu Cao*)
Caulis Polygoni Multiflori (*Ye Jiao Teng*)
Sclerotium Poriae Cocos (*Fu Ling*)

I have already described the functions of each of these medicinals
in the previous chapter when discussing Jean's Chinese
medicinal treatment. These pills are best when taken to prevent
a liver yang headache as opposed to trying to relieve a full-blown
migraine or cluster headache when it is occurring.

Huang Lian Shang Qing Pian (also spelled *Huang Lian Shang Ching Pian)*

These pills treat headache due to wind heat, hyperactivity of liver
yang, and/or liver fire. Their name means Coptis Clear the Upper
Tablets, the upper here referring to the head. Their ingredients
include:

Rhizoma Coptidis Chinensis (*Huang Lian*)
Radix Ligustici Wallichii (*Chuan Xiong*)
Herba Seu Flos Schizonepetae Tenuifoliae (*Jing Jie Sui*)
Radix Ledebouriellae Divaricatae (*Fang Feng*)
Radix Scutellariae Baicalensis (*Huang Qin*)
Radix Platycodi Grandiflori (*Jie Geng*)
Gypsum Fibrosum (*Shi Gao*)
Flos Chrysanthemi Indici (*Ye Ju Hua*)
Radix Angelicae Dahuricae (*Bai Zhi*)
Radix Glycyrrhizae (*Gan Cao*)
Radix Et Rhizoma Rhei (*Da Huang*)

Fructus Viticis (*Man Jing Zi*)
Fructus Forsythiae Suspensae (*Lian Qiao*)
Flos Inulae (*Xuan Fu Hua*)
Cortex Phellodendri (*Huang Bai*)
Herba Menthae Haplocalycis (*Bo He*)
Fructus Gardeniae Jasminoidis (*Shan Zhi Zi*)

These pills are best used if there is also constipation. They should not be used if there is diarrhea or, if they cause diarrhea, they should be stopped. Also, pregnant women should not take these pills. They are not meant for long-term usage since they are bitter and cold and strongly draining.

Long Dan Xie Gan Wan

Long Dan means dragon gall. This is the literal translation of the name of the main ingredient in this formula, Gentiana. *Xie Gan* means to drain the liver, while *wan* simply means pills. This formula is the textbook standard formula for liver fire. The symptoms of liver fire have been given above. The ingredients in this formula include:

Radix Gentianae Scabrae (*Long Dan Cao*)
Fructus Gardeniae Jasminoidis (*Shan Zhi Zi*)
Radix Scutellariae Baicalensis (*Huang Qin*)
Radix Bupleuri (*Chai Hu*)
Caulis Akebiae (*Mu Tong*)
Semen Plantaginis (*Che Qian Zi*)
Rhizoma Alisma (*Ze Xie*)
uncooked Radix Rehmanniae (*Sheng Di*)
Extremitas Radicis Angelicae Sinensis (*Dang Gui Wei*)
Radix Glycyrrhizae (*Gan Cao*)

The ingredients in this formula are very bitter and cold. Therefore, they can easily damage the spleen and stomach. One should only take this formula for a few days. Once the signs of liver fire have abated, its use should be discontinued. If, while taking this formula, you develop diarrhea, stop and consult a professional practitioner. This formula is not meant for long-term usage, but rather for the treatment of acute conditions.

Gui Pi Wan (also spelled Kuei Pi Wan)

Gui means to return or restore, *pi* means the spleen, and *wan* means pills. Therefore, the name of these pills means Restore the Spleen Pills.[9] However, these pills not only supplement the spleen qi but also nourish heart blood and calm the heart spirit. They are the textbook guiding formula for the pattern of heart-spleen dual vacuity. In this case, there are symptoms of spleen qi vacuity, such as fatigue, poor appetite, and cold hands and feet plus symptoms of heart blood vacuity, such as a pale tongue, heart palpitations, and insomnia. This formula is also the standard one for treating heavy or abnormal bleeding due to the spleen not containing and restraining the blood within its vessels. This patent medicine can be combined with *Xiao Yao San* when there is liver depression qi stagnation complicated by heart blood and spleen qi vacuity. It is the most effective Chinese patent medicine for blood vacuity headaches. Its ingredients are:

Radix Astragali Membranacei (*Huang Qi*)
Radix Codonopsitis Pilosulae (*Dang Shen*)
Rhizoma Atractylodis Macrocephalae (*Bai Zhu*)
Sclerotium Parardicis Poriae Cocos (*Fu Shen*)
mix-fried Radix Glycyrrhizae (*Gan Cao*)
Radix Angelicae Sinensis (*Dang Gui*)
Semen Zizyphi Spinosae (*Suan Zao Ren*)
Arillus Euphoriae Longanae (*Long Yan Rou*)
Radix Polygalae Tenuifoliae (*Yuan Zhi*)
Radix Auklandiae Lappae (*Mu Xiang*)

---

[9] When sold as a dried, powdered extract, this formula is called Ginseng & Longan Combination.

Bai Zi Yang Xin Wan

This is another popular Chinese patent pill for a combination of spleen qi vacuity and heart blood vacuity. Its name means Biota Nourish the Heart Pills. They are especially effective when headaches are accompanied by insomnia. Their ingredients are:

Semen Biotae Orientalis (*Bai Zi Ren*)
Fructus Lycii Chinensis (*Gou Qi Zi*)
Radix Scrophulariae Ningpoensis (*Xuan Shen*)
uncooked Radix Rehmanniae (*Sheng Di*)
Tuber Ophiopogonis Japonici (*Mai Dong*)
Radix Angelicae Sinensis (*Dang Gui*)
Sclerotium Poriae Cocos (*Fu Ling*)
Rhizoma Acori Graminei (*Shi Chang Pu*)
Radix Glycyrrhizae (*Gan Cao*)

Er Chen Wan

Er Chen Wan means Two Aged (Ingredients) Pills.[10] This is because, two of its main ingredients are aged before using. This formula is used to transform phlegm and eliminate dampness. It can be added to pretty much any other Chinese patent medicine when there is a heavy component of phlegm and dampness. Its ingredients include:

Rhizoma Pinelliae Ternatae (*Ban Xia*)
Sclerotium Poriae Cocos (*Fu Ling*)
mix-fried Radix Glycyrrhizae (*Gan Cao*)
Pericarpium Citri Reticulatae (*Chen Pi*)
uncooked Rhizoma Zingiberis (*Sheng Jiang*)

All these medicinals either transform phlegm or eliminate dampness.

---

[10] When sold as a dried, powdered extract, this formula is called Citrus & Pinellia Combination.

Liu Wei Di Huang Wan

This formula, whose name means Six Flavors Rehmannia Pills, nourishes liver blood and kidney yin. It is the primary formula to treat symptoms of yin vacuity. Its ingredients are:

cooked Radix Rehmanniae (*Shu Di*)
Fructus Corni Officinalis (*Shan Zhu Yu*)
Radix Dioscoreae Oppositae (*Shan Yao*)
Rhizoma Alismatis (*Ze Xie*)
Sclerotium Poriae Cocos (*Fu Ling*)
Cortex Radicis Moutan (*Dan Pi*)

In a very few people, one of the ingredients, Rehmannia, can cause diarrhea. If these pills cause diarrhea, their use should be stopped immediately.

If there is liver yang hyperactivity but with more pronounced underlying yin vacuity, then one can combine these pills with *Tian Ma Gou Teng Wan*. If there are signs and symptoms of vacuity heat, such as flushed cheeks in the afternoon, low-grade fever, and/or night sweats, then another formula should be used instead. It is made by adding two more ingredients to the above:

Rhizoma Anemarrhenae Aspheloidis (*Zhi Mu*)
Cortex Phellodendri (*Huang Bai*)

This is then called *Zhi Bai Di Huang Wan*, Anemarrhena & Phellodendron Rehmannia Pills.

An Shen Bu Xin Wan

The name of this pill translates as Quiet the Spirit & Supplement the Heart Pills. Though their name includes the word heart, they can be used to treat headache due to yin vacuity. These pills can be used instead of the above formula if *Liu Wei Di Huang Wan* causes diarrhea. Their ingredients include:

Concha Margaritiferae (*Zhen Zhu Mu*)
Caulis Polygoni Multiflori (*Ye Jiao Teng*)
Fructus Ligustri Lucidi (*Nu Zhen Zi*)
Herba Ecliptae Prostratae (*Han Lian Cao*)
Radix Salviae Miltiorrhizae (*Dan Shen*)
Cortex Albizziae Julibrissin (*He Huan Pi*)
Semen Cuscutae Chinensis (*Tu Si Zi*)
Fructus Schisandrae Chinensis (*Wu Wei Zi*)
Rhizoma Acori Graminei (*Shi Chang Pu*)

You Gui Wan

The name of these pills translates as Restore the Right Pills. This is because kidney yang is often referred to as the right kidney. This formula, therefore, is for the treatment of kidney yang vacuity headache. If there are no cold symptoms, such as cold feet, chilly, weak low back, copious, clear, night-time urination, or decreased sexual desire, one should not use this formula. One should also suspend its use if it produces symptoms of evil heat. These might include sores on the tongue or in the mouth, sore throat, fever, or flu-like symptoms. This formula's ingredients include:

cooked Radix Rehmanniae (*Shu Di*)
Radix Lateralis Praeparatus Aconiti Carmichaeli (*Fu Zi*)
Cortex Cinnamomi Cassiae (*Rou Gui*)
Fructus Corni Officinalis (*Shan Zhu Yu*)
Fructus Lycii Chinensis (*Wu Wei Zi*)
Radix Dioscoreae Oppositae (*Shan Yao*)
Cortex Eucommiae Ulmoidis (*Du Zhong*)
Radix Angelicae Sinensis (*Dang Gui*)
Semen Cuscutae Chinensis (*Tu Si Zi*)
Gelatinum Cornu Cervi (*Lu Jiao Jiao*)

Jin Gui Shen Qi Wan

Jin Gui is an allusion to the name of the book this formula is taken from, *The Golden Cabinet*, a book written approximately 250 CE. The rest of the name means kidney qi pills. Along with the preceding formula, this is one of the most famous formulas for supplementing kidney yang in Chinese medicine. The same caveats and cautions apply to its use. Its ingredients consist of:

cooked Radix Rehmanniae (*Shu Di*)
Radix Lateralis Praeparatus Aconiti Carmichaeli (*Fu Zi*)
Cortex Cinnamomi Cassiae (*Rou Gui*)
Fructus Corni Officinalis (*Shan Zhu Yu*)
Radix Dioscoreae Oppositae (*Shan Yao*)
Sclerotium Poriae Cocos (*Fu Ling*)
Rhizoma Alismatis (*Ze Xie*)
Cortex Radicis Moutan (*Dan Pi*)

Bu Zhong Yi Qi Wan

The name of this formula translates as Supplement the Center & Boost the Qi Pills. It strongly supplements spleen vacuity. It is commonly used to treat central qi fall, *i.e.*, prolapse of the stomach, uterus, or rectum due to spleen qi vacuity. However, it is a very complex formula with a very wide range of indications. It supplements the spleen but also courses the liver and rectifies the qi. It is one of the most commonly prescribed of all Chinese herbal formulas and these pills can be combined with a number of others when spleen qi vacuity plays a significant role in someone's condition. Its ingredients are:

Radix Astragali Membranacei (*Huang Qi*)
Radix Panacis Ginseng (*Ren Shen*)
Radix Glycyrrhizae (*Gan Cao*)
Rhizoma Atractylodis Macrocephalae (*Bai Zhu*)
Radix Angelicae Sinensis (*Dang Gui*)
Pericarpium Citri Reticulatae (*Chen Pi*)

Rhizoma Cimicifugae (*Sheng Ma*)
Radix Bupleuri (*Chai Hu)*
Rhizoma Atractylodis Macrocephalae (*Bai Zhu*)

Xue Fu Zhu Yu Wan

The name of these pills in English is Blood Mansion Dispel Stasis Pills. They are a commonly used basic formula for the treatment of blood stasis conditions. They can either be used as the main treatment for a predominately blood stasis pattern, or can be combined with other Chinese patent medicines when blood stasis plays a contributory role. Remember, blood stasis pain is fixed in one spot, is typically severe, and often described as sharp, piercing, or stabbing. One should also remember the saying, "Enduring disease enters the network vessels." This means that chronic diseases are often complicated by blood stasis. The ingredients in this formula consist of:

Semen Pruni Persicae (*Tao Ren*)
Flos Carthami Tinctorii (*Hong Hua*)
Radix Angelicae Sinensis (*Dang Gui*)
Radix Ligustici Wallichii (*Chuan Xiong*)
Radix Rubrus Paeoniae Lactiflorae (*Chi Shao*)
Radix Bupleuri (*Chai Hu*)
Radix Platycodi Grandiflori (*Jie Geng*)
Fructus Citri Aurantii (*Zhi Ke*)
uncooked Radix Rehmanniae (*Sheng Di*)
Radix Glycyrrhizae (*Gan Cao*)

Yan Hu Suo Wan

Called Corydalis Pills in English, this Chinese patent medicine consists of only two ingredients:

Rhizoma Corydalis Yanhusuo (*Yuan Hu Suo*)
Radix Angelicae Dahuricae (*Bai Zhi*)

71

The first ingredient moves the qi and quickens the blood. It is an all-purpose pain-reliever, but is especially effective for pain due to blood stasis. The second ingredient, Angelica, strongly moves the qi. It also tends to rise to the head and treats headache very effectively. These pills can be added to almost any other formula in order to treat the symptoms of a currently occurring, acute headache. They are not meant for long-term use. They do not treat the root of the problem, only the branch symptom of pain. However, that they do effectively.

Bao Ji Wan (also spelled *Po Chai Wan*)

These pills are a very commonly used Chinese patent medicine for food stagnation due to overeating or over-drinking. They consist of a number of ingredients whose action is to disperse food and abduct or lead away stagnation. We often give them out at parties when our guests may have eaten too much, and I have often taken one or two bottles before bed when I have come home from a party or a restaurant where I may have eaten too much. The Chinese name translates as Protect (from) Accumulation Pills. Another similar pill is called **Kang Ning Wan**, Health Stabilizing Pills. These are also sold under the name Curing Pills. The ingredients are a little different, but the action of these two formulas is very similar. Yet another such patent remedy for food stagnation is **Bao He Wan**, Protect Harmony Pills. The ingredients in this last formula are:

Massa Medica Fermentata (*Shen Qu*)
Fructus Crataegi (*Shan Zha*)
Semen Raphani Sativi (*Lai Fu Zi*)
Rhizoma Pinelliae Ternatae (*Ban Xia*)
Sclerotium Poriae Cocos (*Fu Ling*)
Pericarpium Citri Reticulatae (*Chen Pi*)
Fructus Forsythiae Suspensae (*Lian Qiao*)
Fructus Germinatus Hordei Vulgaris (*Mai Ya*)

72

The above are only the most famous and commonly used formulas which are currently available over the counter at American health food stores and at Asian specialty food stores in Asian communities in North America. They can be ordered by phone, fax, or mail from:

Mayway Corp.
1338 Mandela Parkway
Oakland, CA 94607
Tel. 510-208-3113
Orders: 1-800-2-Mayway
Fax: 510-208-3069
Orders by fax: 1-800-909-2828

This company is one of the largest importers and distributors of Chinese herbs and Chinese herbal products in North America and Europe. They have a very nice, easy to use catalog wih easy ordering numbers so you do not need to worry about pronouncing the Chinese names of these formulas. Another company these Chinese patent medicines can be ordered from by phone, mail, or fax is:

Nuherbs Co.
3820 Penniman Ave.
Oakland, CA 94619
Tel. 510-534-4372
Orders: 1-800-233-4307
Fax: 510-534-4384
Orders by fax: 1-800-550-1928

There are many other important formulas used in the professional practice of Chinese medicine. However, for these, you will need to see your local professional practitioner. If you experiment with Chinese herbal patent medicines for your headaches, please be careful. Be sure to follow the six guideposts for assessing the safety of any medications you take.

Six guideposts for assessing any over-the-counter medication

In general, you can tell if *any* medication and treatment are good for you by checking the following six guideposts.

1. Digestion
2. Elimination
3. Energy level

4. Mood
5. Appetite
6. Sleep

If a medication, be it modern Western or traditional Chinese, gets rid of your symptoms and all six of these basic areas of human health improve, then that medicine or treatment is probably ok. However, even if a treatment or medication takes away your major complaint, *if it causes deterioration in any one of these six basic parameters,* then that treatment or medication is probably not ok and is certainly not ok for long term use. When medicines and treatments, even so-called natural, herbal medications, are prescribed based on a person's pattern of disharmony, then there is healing without side effects. According to Chinese medicine, this is the only kind of true healing.

Acupuncture & Moxibustion

Acupuncture is the best known of the various methods of treatment which go to make up Chinese medicine. When the average Westerner thinks of Chinese medicine, they probably first think of acupuncture. In China acupuncture is actually a secondary treatment modality. Most Chinese immediately think of herbal medicine when they think of Chinese medicine. Nevertheless, headaches of all kinds respond very well to correctly prescribed and administered acupuncture.

What is acupuncture?

Acupuncture primarily means the insertion of extremely thin, sterilized, stainless steel needles into specific points on the body where practitioners of Chinese medicine have known for centuries there are special concentrations of qi and blood. Therefore, these points are like switches or circuit breakers for regulating and balancing the flow of qi and blood over the channel and network system we described above.

As we have seen above, all pain in the head is the result of a lack of free flow of the qi and blood in the head. Since acupuncture's forte is the regulation and rectification of the flow of qi, it is an especially good treatment mode for treating headaches. In that case, insertion of acupuncture needles at various points in the body moves the qi which then moves the blood and body fluids. As soon as the flow of qi, blood, and body fluids is normalized, the headache disappears. Remember, "If there is free flow, there is *no pain*." Because acupuncture's effects are immediate, acupuncture is a particularly good first-aid remedy for a head-ache in progress.

As a generic term, acupuncture also includes several other methods of stimulating acupuncture points, thus regulating the flow of qi in the body. The main other modality is moxibustion. This means the warming of acupuncture points mainly by burning dried, aged Oriental mugwort on, near, or over acupuncture points. The purpose of this warming treatment are to 1) even more strongly stimulate the flow of qi and blood, 2) add warmth to areas of the body which are too cold, and 3) add yang qi to the body to supplement a yang qi deficiency. Other acupuncture modalities are to apply suction cups over points, to massage the points, to prick the points to allow a drop or two of blood to exit, to apply Chinese medicinals to the points, to apply magnets to the points, and to stimulate the points by either electricity or laser.

What is a typical acupuncture treatment for headache like?

In China, acupuncture treatments are given every day or every other day, three to five times per week depending on the nature and severity of the condition. In the West however, health care delivery differs greatly from China, making it financially unfeasible for most patients to receive as many treatments per week. Western patients suffering from headaches usually respond well to acupuncture treatments performed twice a week for the first few weeks, followed up with a single treatment once a week for another several weeks. For chronic headaches, after an initial course of 10-12 sessions, it is best to continue acupuncture treatments once a month for several more months. After that, one should get one or two "brush-up" or "booster" treatments whenever they start feeling headachy again.

Based on my clinical experience, if acupuncture is combined with diet and lifestyle changes, Chinese herbs, and a selection of the self-care treatments recommended below, the results will be even quicker and the relief of symptoms even more complete.

When the person comes for their appointment, the practitioner will ask them what their main symptoms are, will typically look at their tongue and its fur, and will feel the pulses at the radial arteries on both wrists. Then, they will ask the patient to lie down on a treatment table and may palpate their abdomen and the zones traversed by the different channels to feel for areas of constriction, tenderness, and blockage. Based on the patient's pattern discrimination, the practitioner will select anywhere from one to eight or nine points to be needled.

The needles used today are ethylene oxide gas sterilized disposable needles. This means that they are used one time and then thrown away, just like a hypodermic syringe in a doctor's office. However, unlike relatively fat hypodermic needles, acupuncture needles are hardly thicker than a strand of hair. The skin over the point is disinfected with alcohol and the needle is quickly and deftly inserted somewhere typically between one quarter and a half inch. In some few cases, a needle may be inserted deeper than that, but most needles are only inserted relatively shallowly.

After the needle has broken the skin, the acupuncturist will usually manipulate the needle in various ways until he or she feels that the qi has "arrived." This refers to a subtle but very real feeling of resistance around the needle. When the qi arrives, the patient will usually feel a mild, dull soreness around the needle, a slight electrical feeling, a heavy feeling, or a numb or tingly feeling. All these mean that the needle has tapped the qi and that treatment will be effective. Once the qi has been tapped, then the practitioner may further adjust the qi flow by manipulating the needle in certain ways, may simply leave the needle in place, usually for 10-20 minutes, or may attach the needle to an electro-acupuncture machine in order to stimulate the point with very mild and gentle electricity. After this, the needles are withdrawn and thrown away. *Thus there is absolutely no chance for infection from another patient.*

How are the points selected?

The points one's acupuncturist chooses to needle each treatment are selected on the basis of Chinese medical theory and the known clinical effects of certain points. Since there are different schools or styles of acupuncture, point selection tends to vary from practitioner to practitioner. However, below is a fairly typical acupuncture treatment for a liver yang hyperactivity pattern headache based on Chinese medical pattern discrimination.

Let's take the case of Jean who we saw before and let's say that she has been able to come in during a migraine attack in progress. Her main complaint is a severe, pounding pain in the left side of her head. We previously established that Jean's Chinese pattern discrimination is liver yang hyperactivity complicated by blood vacuity in turn due to spleen vacuity. However, during the acute episode, we are only going to address the liver yang hyperactivity.

The treatment principles necessary for remedying this case are to soothe the liver and downbear counterflow, subdue yang and stop pain. In order to accomplish these aims, the practitioner might select the following points:

Tai Chong (Liver 3)
He Gu (Large Intestine 4)
Wai Guan (Triple Burner 5)
Zu Lin Qi (Gallbladder 41)
Feng Chi (Gallbladder 20)
Tai Yang (Extra channel point M-HN-9)
A shi points (points of special pain)

In this case, *Tai Chong* courses the liver and resolves depression, moves and rectifies the qi. Rectification of the qi includes the downbearing of upward counterflow.

He Gu is a widely used point with a variety of indications depending on how it is used and with what points it is combined. *Hei Gu* and *Tai Chong* combined are known as "the four gates." They are used to free the flow in the entire body and to promote the upbearing of the clear and downbearing of the turbid by the qi mechanism. When used together, these points have a strong effect in relieving qi stagnation. In addition, *He Gu* is one of the four command points and is one of the two command points for the head and face.

Wai Guan and *Zu Lin Qi* are also a commonly used two point combination. *Wai Guan* is a point on the triple burner channel, while *Zu Lin Qi* is a point on the gallbladder channel. Side of the head headaches mean that the pain is due to a lack of free flow in these two channels which, together, make up the *shao yang*. In this case, the liver is yin, while it is yang which is hyperactive and replete. Therefore, liver yang passes into the yang gallbladder channel with which the liver is paired. Needling these two points on the affected side only helps to free the flow in the *shao yang*. This is a well-known combination for treating side of the head headaches.

Feng Chi is also a *shao yang* gallbladder channel point. It is chosen for the same reason. It frees the flow of the *shao yang* in the affected area. It is combined with *Tai Yang,* one of the most important extra or non-channel points in the body. The name *Tai Yang* means supreme or greatest yang. Therefore, this point is particularly effective in treating hyperactive yang conditions resulting in pathologies manifesting in the head and is even more effective if those pathologies involve the side of the head.

A shi points mean any point which, when pressed, elicits a pain response. In Jean's case, I would needle the places on the side of the head where she said the pain was particularly located. If Jean said that it hurt here, I would needle here. If she said it hurt there, I would needle there. In this manner, I would add somewhere between one and four *a shi* points to the above standardly located points.

Therefore, this combination of points addresses Jean's Chinese pattern discrimination *and* her major complaint of pain. It remedies both the underlying disease mechanism and addresses the key symptom of that mechanism in a very direct and immediate way. Hence it provides symptomatic relief *at the same time* as it corrects the underlying mechanisms of these symptoms.

Does acupuncture hurt?

In Chinese, it is said that acupuncture is *bu tong*, painless. However, most patients will feel soreness, heaviness, electrical tingling, or distention. When done well and sensitively, it should not be sharp, biting, burning, or really painful.

How quickly will I feel the result?

One of the best things about the acupuncture treatment of headache is that its effects are often immediate. Since many of the mechanisms of headache have to do with stuck qi, as soon as the qi is made to flow, the symptoms disappear. Therefore, many patients begin to feel better after the very first treatment.

In addition, because irritability and nervous tension are also mostly due to liver depression qi stagnation, most people will feel an immediate relief of irritability and tension while still on the table. Typically, one will feel a pronounced tranquility and relaxation within five to 10 minutes of the insertion of the needles. Many patients do drop off to sleep for a few minutes while the needles are in place.

Who should get acupuncture?

Since most professional practitioners in the West are legally entitled to practice under various acupuncture laws, most acupuncturists will routinely do acupuncture on every patient. Since acupuncture's effects on headache are usually relatively immediate, this is usually a good thing for sufferers of headache. However, acupuncture is particularly effective for liver yang hyperactivity, liver fire exuberance, phlegm dampness, food retention, roundworm, and blood stasis patterns of headache.

When a person's headaches mostly have to do with qi vacuity, blood vacuity, yin or yang vacuity, then acupuncture is most effective when combined with internally administered Chinese herbal medicinals. Although moxibustion can add yang qi to the body, acupuncture needles cannot add qi, blood, or yin to a body in short supply of these. The best acupuncture can do in these cases is to stimulate the various viscera and bowels which engender and transform the qi, blood, and yin. Chinese herbs, on the other hand, can directly introduce qi, blood, and yin into the body, thus supplementing vacuities and insufficiencies of these. In cases of headache, where qi, blood, and yin vacuities are pronounced, one should use acupuncture in combination with Chinese medicinals.

Ear acupuncture

Acupuncturists believe there is a map of the entire body in the ear and that by stimulating the corresponding points in the ear, one can remedy those areas and functions of the body. Therefore, many acupuncturists will not only needle points on the body at large but also select one or more points on the ear. In terms of headache, there are points which correspond to the head as well as points which correspond to the liver, gallbladder, spleen, stomach, and kidneys, all the viscera and bowels which participate in the various Chinese disease mechanisms of headache. Other points, such as Spirit Gate, Sympathetic Point, Brain Point, and Subcortex Point are very effective for relieving stress and generally calming the nervous system.

The nice thing about ear acupuncture points is that one can use tiny "press needles" which are shaped like miniature thumbtacks. These are pressed into the points, covered with adhesive tape, and left in place for five to seven days. This method can provide continuous treatment between regularly scheduled office visits. Thus ear acupuncture is a nice way of extending the duration of an acupuncture treatment. In addition, these ear points can also be stimulated with small metal pellets, radish seeds, or tiny magnets, thus getting the benefits of stimulating these points without having to insert actual needles.

The Three Free Therapies

Although one can experiment cautiously with Chinese herbal medicinals, one cannot really do acupuncture on oneself. Therefore, Chinese herbal medicine and acupuncture and its related modalities mostly require the aid of a professional practitioner. However, there are three free therapies which are crucial to treating headaches which are in turn due to either stress or faulty diet. These are diet, exercise, and deep relaxation. Only you can take care of these three factors in your health!

Diet

In Chinese medicine, the function of the spleen and stomach are likened to a pot on a stove or still. The stomach receives the foods and liquids which then "rotten and ripen" like a mash in a fermentation vat. The spleen then cooks this mash and drives off (*i.e.,* transforms and upbears) the pure part. This pure part collects in the lungs to become the qi and in the heart to become the blood. In addition, Chinese medicine characterizes this transformation as a process of yang qi transforming yin substance. All the principles of Chinese dietary therapy, including what persons with headaches should and should not eat, are derived from these basic "facts."

We have already seen that the spleen is the root of qi and blood engenderment and transformation. Likewise, the spleen is in charge of the movement and transformation of body fluids. Based on these facts, a healthy, strong spleen prevents and treats headaches in several ways. First of all, a strong spleen is one way of keeping the liver in check. It is said that once the liver is diseased, the next most likely viscus to be affected is the spleen. Therefore, it is also said that, "When the liver is diseased, first treat the spleen." Secondly, if the spleen is healthy and strong, it will create sufficient qi to push the blood and move body fluids. Therefore, a sufficiency of pushing or moving spleen qi helps counterbalance or control any tendency to either bood stasis or phlegm dampness. Third, the spleen is the root of blood production. Therefore, a healthy spleen insures there is sufficient blood to A) nourish and soften the liver, and B) fill the brain. In addition, excess blood not consumed by life's activities is converted into yin essence to be stored in the kidneys. Thus supplementing the spleen in order to nourish the blood is an indirect way of enriching and supplementing kidney yin. Excess qi is turned into yang essence. Thus supplementing the spleen in order to boost the qi is an indirect way of invigorating and supplementing kidney yang.

Therefore, when it comes to Chinese dietary therapy and headaches, the fundamental principle is to avoid foods which damage the spleen. Such foods also typically produce dampness and phlegm.

Foods which damage the spleen

In terms of foods which damage the spleen, Chinese medicine begins with uncooked, chilled foods. If the process of digestion is likened to cooking, then cooking is nothing other than predigestion outside of the body. In Chinese medicine, it is a given that the overwhelming majority of all food should be cooked, i.e., predigested. Although cooking may destroy some vital nutrients (in Chinese, qi), cooking does render the remaining nutrients much more easily assimilable. Therefore, even though some nutrients have been lost, the net absorption of nutrients is greater with cooked foods than raw. Further, eating raw foods makes the spleen work harder and thus wears the spleen out more quickly. If one's spleen is very robust, eating uncooked, raw foods may not be so damaging, but specially for women their spleens are already weak because of their monthly menses overtaxing the spleen *vis à vis* blood production. It is also a fact of life that the spleen typically becomes weak with age.

More importantly, chilled foods directly damage the spleen. Chilled, frozen foods and drinks neutralize the spleen's yang qi. The process of digestion is the process of turning all foods and drinks to 100° Fahrenheit soup within the stomach so that it may undergo distillation. If the spleen expends too much yang qi just warming the food up, then it will become damaged and weak. Therefore, all foods and liquids should be eaten and drunk at room temperature at the least and better at body temperature. The more signs and symptoms of spleen vacuity a person presents, such as fatigue, chronically loose stools, undigested food in the stools, cold hands and feet, dizziness on standing up, and aversion to cold, the more closely he or she should avoid uncooked, chilled foods and drinks.

In addition, sugars and sweets directly damage the spleen. This is because sweet is the flavor which inherently "gathers" in the spleen. It is also an inherently dampening flavor according to Chinese medicine. This means that the body engenders or secretes fluids which gather and collect, transforming into dampness, in response to foods with an excessively sweet flavor. In Chinese medicine, it is said that the spleen is averse to dampness. Dampness is yin and controls or checks yang qi. The spleen's function is based on the transformative and transporting functions of yang qi. Therefore, anything which is excessively dampening can damage the spleen. The sweeter a food is, the more dampening and, therefore, more damaging it is to the spleen.

Another food which is dampening and, therefore, damaging to the spleen is what Chinese doctors call "sodden wheat foods." This means flour products such as bread and noodles. Wheat (as opposed to rice) is damp by nature. When wheat is steamed, yeasted, and/or refined, it becomes even more dampening. In addition, all oils and fats are damp by nature and, hence, may damage the spleen. The more oily or greasy a food is, the worse it is for the spleen. Because milk contains a lot of fat, dairy products are another spleen-damaging, dampness-engendering food. This includes milk, butter, and cheese.

If we put this all together, then ice cream is just about the worst thing a person with a weak, damp spleen could eat. Ice cream is chilled, it is intensely sweet, and it is filled with fat. Therefore, it is a triple whammy when it comes to damaging the spleen. Likewise, pasta smothered in tomato sauce and cheese is a recipe for disaster. Pasta made from wheat flour is dampening, tomatoes are dampening, and cheese is dampening. In addition, what many people don't know is that a glass of fruit juice contains as much sugar as a candy bar, and, therefore, is also very damaging to the spleen and damp-engendering.

Below is a list of specific Western foods which are either uncooked, chilled, too sweet, or too dampening and thus damaging to the spleen. Persons with headaches due to or involving qi vacuity, blood vacuity, phlegm dampness, or food stagnation should minimize or avoid these proportional to how weak and damp their spleen is.

Ice cream
Sugar
Candy, especially chocolate
Milk
Butter
Cheese
Margarine
Yogurt
Raw salads
Fruit juices

Juicy, sweet fruits, such as oranges, peaches, strawberries, and tomatoes
Fatty meats
Fried foods
Refined flour products
Yeasted bread
Nuts
Alcohol (which is essentially sugar)

If the spleen is weak and wet, one should also not eat too much at any one time. A weak spleen can be overwhelmed by a large meal, especially if any of the food is hard-to-digest. This then results in food stagnation which only impedes the free flow of qi all the more and further damages the spleen.

A clear, bland diet

In Chinese medicine, the best diet for the spleen and, therefore, by extension for most humans, is what is called a "clear, bland diet." This is a diet high in complex carbohydrates such as unrefined grains, especially rice and beans. It is a diet which is high in *lightly cooked* vegetables. It is a diet which is low in fatty meats, oily, greasy, fried foods, and very sweet foods. However, it is not a completely vegetarian diet. Most people, in my experience should eat one to two ounces of various types of meat two to four times per week. This animal flesh may be the highly popular but over touted chicken and fish, but should also include some lean beef, pork, and lamb. Some fresh or cooked fruits may be eaten, but fruit juices should be avoided. In addition, women especially should make an effort to include tofu and tempeh, two soy foods now commonly available in North American grocery food stores.

If the spleen is weak, then one should eat several smaller meals than one or two large meals. In addition, because rice is 1) neutral in temperature, 2) it fortifies the spleen and supplements the qi, and 3) it eliminates dampness, rice should be the main or staple grain in the diet.

A few problem foods

Coffee
There are a few "problem" foods which deserve special mention. The first of these is coffee. Many people crave coffee for two reasons. First, coffee moves stuck qi. Therefore, if a person

suffers from liver depression qi stagnation, temporarily coffee will make them feel like their qi is flowing. Secondly, coffee transforms essence into qi and makes that qi temporarily available to the body. Therefore, people who suffer from spleen and/or kidney vacuity fatigue will get a temporary lift from coffee. They will feel like they have energy. However, once this energy is used up, they are left with a negative deficit. The coffee has transformed some of the essence stored in the kidneys into qi. This qi has been used, and now there is less stored essence. Since the blood and essence share a common source, coffee drinking may cause or ultimately worsen headaches associated with blood or kidney vacuities. Tea has a similar effect as coffee in that it transforms yin essence into yang qi and liberates that upward and outward through the body. However, the caffeine in black tea is usually only half as strong as in coffee.

Chocolate

Another problem food is chocolate. Chocolate is a combination of oil, sugar, and cocoa. We have seen that both oil and sugar are dampening and damaging to the spleen. Temporarily, the sugar will boost the spleen qi, but ultimately it will result in "sugar blues" or a hypoglycemic let-down. Cocoa stirs the life gate fire. The life gate fire is another name for kidney yang or kidney fire, and kidney fire is the source of sexual energy and desire. It is said that chocolate is the food of love, and from the Chinese medical point of view, that is true. Since chocolate stimulates kidney fire at the same time as it temporarily boosts the spleen, it does give one a rush of yang qi. In addition, this rush of yang qi does move depression and stagnation, at least short-term. So it makes sense that some people with liver depression, spleen vacuity, and kidney yang debility might crave chocolate. However, kidney yang is the source of liver yang. Therefore, chocolate can lead directly to upward flaring of liver fire or hyperactivity of liver yang.

Alcohol

Alcohol is both damp and hot according to Chinese medical theory. Hence, in English it is referred to as "fire water." It strongly moves the qi and blood. Therefore, persons with liver depression qi stagnation will feel temporarily better from drinking alcohol. However, the sugar in alcohol damages the spleen and engenders dampness which "gums up the works," while the heat (yang) in alcohol can waste the blood (yin) and aggravate or inflame depressive liver heat and/or hyperactive liver yang.

Hot, peppery foods

Spicy, peppery, "hot" foods also move the qi, thereby giving some temporary relief to liver depression qi stagnation. However, like alcohol, the heat in spicy hot foods wastes the blood and can inflame yang.

Sour foods

In Chinese medicine, the sour flavor is inherently astringing and constricting. Therefore, people with liver depression qi stagnation should be careful not to use vinegar and other intensely sour foods. Such sour flavored foods will only aggravate the qi stagnation by astringing and restricting the qi and blood all the more. This is also why sweet and sour foods, such as orange juice and tomatoes are particularly bad for people with liver depression and spleen vacuity. The sour flavor astringes and constricts the qi, while the sweet flavor damages the spleen and engenders dampness.

Foods which help nourish the blood

Qi & *Wei*

According to Chinese dietary therapy, all foods contain varying proportions of qi and *wei*. Qi means the ability to catalyze or promote yang function, while *wei* (literally meaning flavor) refers to a food's ability to nourish or construct yin substance. Since blood is relatively yin compared to qi being yang, a certain amount of food high in *wei* is necessary for a person to engender and transform blood. Foods which are high in *wei* as compared to qi are those which tend to be heavy, dense, greasy or oily, meaty or bloody. All animal products contain more *wei* than vegetable products. At the same time, black beans or, even better, black soybeans contain more *wei* than celery or lettuce.

When people suffer from headaches due to blood vacuity failing to nourish the brain, they usually need to eat slightly more foods high in *wei*. This includes animal proteins and products, such as meat and eggs. It is said that flesh foods are very "compassionate" to the human body. This word recognizes the fact that the animal's life has had to be sacrificed to produce this type of food. It also recognizes that, because such food is so close to the human body itself, it is especially nutritious. Therefore, when people suffer from blood vacuity headaches, eating some animal products usually is helpful and sometimes is down right necessary.

Animal foods vs. vegetarianism

Based on my many years of clinical experience, I have seen many Westerners adhering to a strict vegetarian diet develop, after several years, blood or yin vacuity patterns. This is especially the case in women who lose blood every month and must build babies out of the blood and yin essence. When women who are strict vegetarians come to me with various complaints, if they present the signs and symptoms of blood vacuity, such as a fat, pale tongue, pale face, pale nails, and pale lips, heart palpitations, insomnia, and fatigue with a fine, forceless pulse, I typically recommend that they include a little animal food in their diet. In such cases, they commonly report to me how much better they feel immediately—how much more energy they have.

The downside of eating meat—besides the ethical issues—are that foods which are high in *wei* also tend to be harder to digest and to engender phlegm and dampness. Therefore, such foods should only be eaten in very small amounts at any one time. In addition, the weaker the person's spleen or the more phlegm and dampness they already have, the less such foods they should eat.

Remember above we said that the process of digestion first consisted of turning the food and drink ingested into 100° soup in the stomach. Therefore, soups and broths made out of animal flesh are the easiest and most digestible way of adding some animal-quality *wei* to a person's diet. When eating flesh itself, this should probably be limited to only one to two ounces per serving and only three or four such servings per week. According to Chinese dietary theory, the best foods for engendering and transforming blood and yin essence (but also the hardest to digest) are organ meats and red or dark meats. This includes beef, buffalo, venison, and lamb and dark meat from chicken, turkey, goose, and duck. White meat fish and white meat fowl are less effective for building blood. However, white meat pork is also ok, as is ham.

One good recipe for adding more digestible *wei* to the diet of a person who is blood vacuous is to take a marrow bone and boil this with some cut vegetables, especially root vegetables, and black beans or black soybeans. Such a marrow bone, black bean, and vegetable soup is easy to digest and yet rich in *wei*.

In the following chapter, the reader will find some specific recipes combining Chinese herbs and foods to treat or prevent various patterns of headache.

Some last words on diet

In conclusion, Western patients are always asking me what they should eat in order to cure their disease. However, when it comes to diet, sad to say, the issue is not so much what to eat as what not to eat. Diet most definitely plays a major role in the cause and perpetuation of many people's headaches, but, except in the case of vegetarians suffering from blood or yin vacuities, the issue is mainly what to avoid or minimize, not what to eat. Most of us know that coffee, chocolate, sugars and sweets, oils and fats, and alcohol are not good for us. Most of us know that we should be eating more complex carbohydrates and freshly cooked vegetables and less fatty meats. However, it's one thing to know these things and another to follow what we know.

To be perfectly honest, a clear bland diet à la Chinese medicine is not the most exciting diet in the world. It is the traditional diet of most lower and lower middle class peoples around the world living in temperate climates. It is the traditional diet of most of my readers' great grandparents. The point I am making here is that our modern Western diet which is high in oils and fats, high in sugars and sweets, high in animal proteins, and proportionally high in uncooked, chilled foods and drinks is a relatively recent aberration, and you can't fool Mother Nature.

When one switches to the clear, bland diet of Chinese medicine, at first one may suffer from cravings for more "flavorful" food. These cravings are, in many cases, actually associated with food "allergies." In other words, we may crave what is actually not good for us similar to a drunk's craving alcohol. After a few days, these cravings tend to disappear and we may be amazed that we don't miss some of our convenience or "comfort" foods as much as we thought we would. If one has been addicted to a food like sugar for many years, it does not take much to "fall off the wagon" and be addicted again. Therefore, perseverance is the key to long-term success. As the Chinese say, a million is made up of nothing but lots of ones, and a bucket is quickly filled by steady drips and drops.

Exercise

Exercise is the second of what I call the three free therapies. According to Chinese medicine, regular and adequate exercise has two basic benefits. First, exercise promotes the movement of the qi and quickening of the blood. Since all headaches involve a lack of free flow, it is obvious that exercise is an important therapy for moving the qi and quickening the blood. Secondly, exercise benefits the spleen. The spleen's movement and transportation of the digestate is dependent upon the qi mechanism. The qi mechanism describes the function of the qi in upbearing the pure and downbearing the turbid parts of digestion. For the qi mechanism to function properly, the qi must be flowing normally and freely. Since exercise moves and rectifies the qi, it also helps regulate and rectify the qi mechanism. This then results in the spleen's movement and transportation of foods and liquids and its subsequent engendering and transforming of the qi and blood. Because spleen qi vacuity and dampness accumulation typically complicate many people's headaches and because a healthy spleen checks and controls a depressed or hyperactive liver, exercise treats one or the other commonly encountered disease mechanisms in the majority of Westerner's suffering from headache. Therefore, it is easy to see that regular, adequate exercise is a vitally important component of any person's regime for either preventing or treating depression.

What kind of exercise is best for headaches?

Aerobics

In my experience, I find aerobic exercise to be the most beneficial for most people with headaches. By aerobic exercise, I mean *any physical activity which raises one's heartbeat 80% above their normal resting rate and keeps it there for at least 20 minutes*. To calculate your normal resting heart rate, place your fingers over the pulsing artery on the front side of your neck. Count the beats for 15 seconds and then multiply by four. This gives you your beats per minute or BPM. Now multiply your BPM by 0.8. Take the resulting number and add it to your resting BPM. This gives you your aerobic threshold of BPM. Next engage in any physical activity you like. After you have been exercising for five minutes, take your pulse for 15 seconds once again at the artery on the front side of your throat. Again multiply the resulting count by four and this tells you your current BPM. If this number is less than your aerobic threshold BPM, then you know you need to exercise harder or faster. Once you get your heart rate up to your aerobic threshold, then you need to keep exercising at the same level of intensity for at least 20 minutes. In order to insure that one is keeping their heartbeat high enough for long enough, one should recount their pulse every five minutes or so.

Depending on one's age and physical condition, different people will have to exercise harder to reach their aerobic threshold than others. For some, simply walking briskly will raise their heartbeat 80% above their resting rate. For others, they will need to do calisthenics, running, swimming, racket ball, or some other, more strenuous exercise. It really does not matter what the exercise is as long as it raises your heartbeat 80% above your resting rate and keeps it there for 20 minutes. However, there are two other criteria that should be met. One, the exercise should be something that is not too boring. If it is too boring, then you may have a hard time keeping up your schedule. Since most people do find aerobic exercises such as running, stationary bicycles, and stair-steppers boring, it is good to listen to music or watch TV in order to distract your mind from the tedium. Secondly, the type of exercise should not cause any damage to any parts of the body. For instance, running on pavement may cause knee problems for some people. Therefore, you should pick a type of exercise you enjoy but also one which will not cause any problems.

When doing aerobic exercise, it is best to exercise either every day or every other day. If one does not do their aerobics at least once every 72 hours, then its cumulative effects will not be as great. Therefore, I recommend my patients with headaches to do some sort of aerobic exercises every day or every other day, three to four times per week *at least*. The good news is that there is no real need to exercise more than 30 minutes at any one time. Forty-five minutes per session is not going to be all that much better than 25 minutes per session. And 25 minutes four times per week is very much better than one hour once a week.

Too much exercise

While the vast majority of people with depression will benefit from more exercise, there are a few who actually need less physical activity. As we have seen, all stirring or activity entails a consumption of yin by yang. If a person is either constitutionally yin vacuous or, due to some circumstance, like aging, enduring disease, extreme blood loss, excessive births, or lactation, has become yin vacuous, then too much exercise or physical activity can worsen that yin vacuity. This is mostly seen in women with thin bodily constitutions who over-exercise, such as professional athletes, or in women who suffer from anorexia and bulemia.

Body fat in Chinese medicine is nothing other than yin. Therefore, people who are very thinly built tend to have less yin to begin with. If, through exercise, one reduces their body fat even more, it may become so insufficient that yin can no longer control yang. In women, such an insufficiency of yin blood due to overconsumption in turn due to too much exercise usually manifests itself first as cessation of menstruation or amenorrhea. However, it is also possible for drug use, especially types of "speed", or anorexia and bulemia to also result in an overconsumption of yin leading to amenorrhea on the one hand and increased mental agitation and insomnia on the other. Here I am using the term bulemia as binging and purging, *i.e.*, eating but vomiting back up whatever has been ingested. Although the woman may be eating, often she still is not getting sufficient yin nourishment. It is also not uncommon to find an attraction to speed, a tendency to over-exercise, and a tendency to anorexia all in the same woman.

In such women, it may be necessary to actually curtail the amount of exercise they are getting. One knows if the amount of exercise they are getting is a good amount if they feel refreshed and invigorated a couple of hours after the exercise is over. If, on the other hand, one feels even more fatigued or feels even more

95

nervous and jittery, or if exercise during the day leads to night sweats and insomnia at night, then one should consider actually doing less exercise.

Deep relaxation

As we have seen above, headaches are commonly associated with hyperactive liver yang counterflowing upward, and hyperactive liver yang typically evolves from long-term or severe liver depression qi stagnation. If liver depression endures or is severe, it typically transforms into heat or fire. Heat or fire being yang, consume and exhaust yin and blood. Thus yang qi moves frenetically upward to crash into the bony box of the skull. Therefore, liver depression qi stagnation is often at the root of headache. In Chinese medicine, liver depression comes from not fulfilling all one's desires. But no adult living in a civilized society can fulfill all their desires. This is why a certain amount of liver depression is endemic among adults. When our desires are frustrated, our qi becomes depressed. This then creates emotional depression and easy anger or irritability. In Chinese medicine, anger is nothing other than the venting of pent up qi in the liver. When qi becomes depressed in the liver, it accumulates like hot air in a balloon. Eventually, that hot, depressed, angry qi has to go somewhere. So when there is a little more frustration or stress, then this angry qi in the liver vents itself upward as irritability, anger, shouting, or nasty words, or as headache, dizziness, vertigo, and facial nervous tics. In Chinese medicine, it is a basic statement of fact that, "Anger results in the qi ascending."

Essentially, this type of anger and irritability are due to a maladaptive coping response that is typically learned at a young age. When we feel frustrated or stressed, stymied by or angry about something, most of us tense our muscles and especially the muscles in our upper back and shoulders, neck, and jaws. At the same time, many of us will hold our breaths. In Chinese medicine, the sinews are governed by the liver. This tensing of the muscles, *i.e.*, the sinews, constricts the flow of qi in the channels and network vessels. Since it is the liver which is responsible for the coursing and discharging of this qi, such tensing of the sinews leads to liver depression qi stagnation. Because the lungs govern the downward spreading and movement of the qi, holding our breath due to stress or frustration only worsens this tendency of the qi not to move and, therefore, to become depressed in the Chinese medical idea of the liver.

Therefore, deep relaxation is the third of the three free therapies. For deep relaxation to be therapeutic medically, it needs to be more than just mental equilibrium. It needs to be somatic or bodily relaxation as well as mental repose. Most of us no longer recognize that every thought we think and feeling we feel is actually a felt physical sensation somewhere in our body. The words we use to describe emotions are all abstract nouns, such as anger, depression, sadness, and melancholy. However, in Chinese medicine, *every emotion is associated with a change in the direction or flow of qi.* As we have said above, anger makes the qi move upward. Fear, on the other hand, makes the qi move downward. Therefore, anger "makes our gorge rise" or "blows our top", while fear may cause a "sinking feeling" or make us "pee in our pants." These colloquial expressions are all based on the age-old wisdom that all thoughts and emotions are not just mental but also bodily events. This is why it is not just enough to clear one's mind. Clearing one's mind is good, but for really marked therapeutic results, it is even better if one clears one's mind at the same time as relaxing every muscle in the body as well as the breath.

Guided deep relaxation tapes

A very efficient and effective way to practice such mental and physical deep relaxation is to do a daily, guided, progressive, deep relaxation audiotape. Guided means that a narrator on the tape leads one through the process of deep relaxation. Such tapes are progressive since they lead one through the body in a progressive manner, first relaxing one body part and then moving on to another. For instance, the narrator may say something to the effect that, as you exhale, you should feel your forehead get heavy and relaxed, softening and expanding, becoming warm and heavy. As you exhale again, now feel your cheeks get heavy and relaxed, softening and expanding, becoming warm and heavy. Breathe in and breathe out, letting your breath go without hindrance or hesitation. Breathing out, now feel your jaw muscles become heavy and relaxed, expanding and softening, becoming warm and heavy, etc., etc. throughout the entire body until one comes to the bottoms of one's feet.

There are innumerable such tapes on the market. These are usually sold in health food stores, New Age music and supply stores, or in bookstores with a good selection of New Age books. Over the years of suggesting this method of deep relaxation to my patients, I have found that each patient will have his or her own preferences in terms of the type of voice, male or female, the choice of words and imagery, whether there is background music or not, and the actual pace of the progression through the body, some narrators speaking a slightly different rate and rhythm. Therefore, I suggest listening to and even purchasing more than one such tape. One should find a tape which they like and can listen to without internal criticism or comment, going along like a cloud in the sky as the narrator's voice blows away all your mental and bodily stress and tension. If one has more than one tape, one can also switch every now and again from tape to tape so as not to become bored with the process or desensitized to the instructions.

Key things to look for in a good relaxation tape

In order to get the full therapeutic effect of such deep relaxation tapes, there are several key things to check for. First, be sure that the tape is a guided tape and not a subliminal relaxation tape. Subliminal tapes usually have music and any instructions to relax are given so quietly that they are not consciously heard. Although such tapes can help you feel relaxed when you do them, ultimately they do not teach you how to relax as a skill which can be consciously practiced and refined. Secondly, make sure the tape starts from the top of the body and works downward. Remember, anger makes the qi go upward in the body, and people with irritability and easy anger due to liver depression qi stagnation already have too much qi rising upward in their bodies. Such depressed qi typically needs not only to be moved but also downborne. Third, make sure the tape instructs you to relax your physical body. If you do not relax all your muscles or sinews, the qi cannot flow freely and the liver cannot be coursed. Depression is not resolved, and there will not be the same medically therapeutic effect. And lastly, be sure the tape instructs you to let your breath go with each exhalation. One of the symptoms of liver depression is a stuffy feeling in the chest which we then unconsciously try to relieve by sighing. Letting each exhalation go completely helps the lungs push the qi downward. This allows the lungs to control the liver at the same time as it downbears upwardly counterflowing angry liver qi.

The importance of daily practice

I was once taken on a field trip to a hospital clinic where they were using deep relaxation as a therapy with patients with high blood pressure, heart disease, stroke, migraines, and insomnia. The doctors at this clinic showed us various graphs plotting their research data on how such daily, progressive deep relaxation can regulate the blood pressure and body temperature and improve the appetite, digestion, elimination, sleep, energy, and mood. One of the things they said has stuck with me for 15 years: "Small results in 100 days, big results in 1,000." This means that if one does such daily, progressive deep relaxation *every single day for 100 days*, one will definitely experience certain results. What are these "small" results? These small results are improvements in all the parameters listed above: blood pressure, body temperature, appetite, digestion, elimination, sleep, energy, and mood. If these are "small" results, then what are the "big" results experienced in 1,000 days of practice? The "big" results are a change in how one reacts to stress—in other words, a change in one's very personality or character.

What these doctors in Shanghai stressed and what I have also experienced both personally and with my patients is that the effects of this relaxation are cumulative. This means that the longer one can practice this routine on a consistent daily basis, the greater and more lasting the effects will be.

It is vitally important to do such daily, guided, progressive deep relaxation every single day, day in and day out for a solid three months at least and for a continuous three years at best. If one does such progressive, somatic deep relaxation every day, *one will see every parameter or measurement of health and well-being improve.* If one does this kind of deep relaxation only sporadically, missing a day here and there, it will feel good when you do it, but it will not have the marked, cumulative therapeutic effects it can. Therefore, perseverance is the real key to getting the benefits of deep relaxation.

The real test

Doing such a daily deep relaxation regime is like hitting tennis balls against a wall or hitting a bucket of balls at a driving range. It is only practice; it is not the real game itself. Doing a daily deep relaxation regime is not only in order to relieve one's immediate stress and strain. It is to learn a new skill, a new way to react to stress. The ultimate goal is to learn how to breathe out and immediately relax all one's muscles in the body in reaction to stress, rather than the common but unhealthy maladaptation to stress of holding one's breath and tensing one's muscles. By doing such deep relaxation day after day, one learns how to relax any and every muscle in the body quickly and efficiently. Then,

100

as soon as one recognizes they are feeling frustrated, stressed out, or uptight, they can immediately remedy those feelings at the same time as coursing their liver and rectifying their qi. This is the real test, the game of life. "Small results in 100 days, big results in 1,000."

Simple Home Remedies for Headaches

Although faulty diet, lack of adequate exercise, and too much stress are the most significant contributing factors to most people's headaches according to Chinese medicine and, therefore, diet, exercise, and deep relaxation are the most important parts of every person's treatment and prevention of headache, there are a number of simple Chinese home remedies to help cure or relieve the symptoms of headache.

Chinese aromatherapy

In Chinese medicine, the qi is seen as a type of wind or vapor. The Chinese character for qi shows wind blowing over a rice field. In addition, smells are often referred to as a thing's qi. Therefore, there is a close relationship between smells carried through the air and the flow of qi in a person's body. Although aromatherapy has not been a major part of professionally practiced Chinese medicine for almost a thousand years, there is a simple aromatherapy treatment which one can do at home which can help alleviate irritability, depression, nervousness, anxiety, and insomnia.

In Chinese, *Chen Xiang* means "sinking fragrance." It is the name of Lignum Aquilariae Agallochae or Eaglewood. This is a frequent ingredient in Asian incense formulas. In Chinese medicine, Aquilaria is classified as a qi-rectifying medicinal. When used as a boiled decoction or "tea", Aquilaria moves the qi and stops pain, downbears upward counterflow and regulates the middle (*i.e.*, the spleen and stomach), and promotes the kidneys'

103

grasping of the qi sent down by the lungs. I believe that the word sinking in this herb's name refers to this medicinal's downbearing of upwardly counterflowing qi. Such upwardly counterflowing eventually must accumulate in the heart, disturbing and causing restlessness of the heart spirit. When this medicinal wood is burnt and its smoke is inhaled as a medicinal incense, its downbearing and spirit-calming function is emphasized.

One can buy Aquilaria or *Chen Xiang* from Chinese herb stores in Chinatowns, Japantowns, or Koreatowns in major urban areas. One can also buy it from Chinese medical practitioners who have their own pharmacies. (See below for addresses, phone numbers, and fax numbers for companies selling Chinese herbs by mail.) It is best to use the powdered variety. However, powder may be made by putting a small piece of this aromatic wood in a coffee grinder. It is also ok to use small bits of the wood if powder is not available. Next one needs to buy a roll of incense charcoals. Place one charcoal in a non-flammable dish and light it with a match. Then sprinkle a few pinches of Aquilaria powder on the lit charcoal. As the smoke rises, breathe in deeply. This can be done on a regular basis one or more times per day on an as-needed basis by those suffering from restlessness, nervousness, anxiety, and irritability. For those who are experiencing on-going stress, one can do this "treatment" on a regular basis at least three times per week.

This Chinese aromatherapy with Lignum Aquilariae Agallochae is very cheap and effective. I know of no side effects or contraindications.

Inhalation therapy

Somewhat similar to aromatherapy is inhalation therapy. However, the preceding aromatherapy regime is meant to primarily treat liver depression qi stagnation, not headaches per se. The following inhalation therapy is meant to actually relieve the symptoms of pain in the head while they are occurring. In other words, this is a first-aid treatment for headaches. But before one can use it, one first has to prepare the medicinal powder that you are going to inhale. Therefore, begin by grinding the following Chinese medicinals into fine powder:

Radix Ligustici Wallichii (*Chuan Xiong*), 1 part
Herba Asari Cum Radice (*Xi Xin*), ½ part
Radix Et Rhizoma Notopterygii (*Qiang Huo*), 1 part
Flos Camelliae Sinensis (*Cha Ye*), 1 part
Herba Seu Flos Schizonepetae Tenuifoliae (*Jing Jie Sui*), 1 part
Radix Platycodi Grandiflori (*Jie Geng*), 1 part
Radix Ledebouriellae Divaricatae (*Fang Feng*), 1 part
Radix Angelicae Dahuricae (*Bai Zhi*), 1 part
Herba Menthae Haplocalycis (*Bo He*), 1 part

At the time of pain, inhale one tenth of one gram of this powder through the nostril on the affected side and then exhale through the mouth. If both sides are affected, then inhale one tenth of one gram through each nostril. One can repeat this at intervals of 15 minutes or more. However, do not continue with this therapy if A) it causes any difficulty breathing, or B) it causes pain or bleeding from the nose or sinus cavities. In most cases, this inhalant powder actually helps treat sinus infections. See below for information on how to order these Chinese herbs.

Chinese herbal pillow

The following recipe is for a Chinese herbal pillow. It can be used for those suffering from headaches of various patterns but

105

especially those associated with blood stasis. The ingredients in this formula quicken the blood and dispel stasis. Grind the following medicinals into powder and sew them into a small, flat cotton bag just big enough to lay the head upon:

Radix Angelicae Sinensis (*Dang Gui*), 2 parts
Radix Et Rhizoma Notopterygii (*Qiang Huo*), 1 part
Radix Ligustici Wallichii (*Chuan Xiong*), 2 parts
Radix Lateralis Praeparatus Aconiti Carmichaeli (*Fu Zi*), ½ part
Radix Aconiti (*Chuan Wu*), ½ part
Radix Et Rhizoma Ligustici Chinensis (*Gao Ben*), 1 part
Radix Rubrus Paeoniae Lactiflorae (*Chi Shao*), 1 part
Flos Carthami Tinctorii (*Hong Hua*), 1 part
Lumbricus (*Di Long*), 1 part
Sanguis Draconis (*Xue Jie*), 1 part
Rhizoma Acori Graminei (*Shi Chang Pu*), 1 part
Medulla Junci (*Deng Xin Cao*), 1 part
Herba Asari Cum Radice (*Xi Xin*), ½ part
Ramulus Cinnamomi Cassiae (*Gui Zhi*), 1 part
Radix Salviae Miltiorrhizae (*Dan Shen*), 1 part
Radix Ledebouriellae Divaricatae (*Fang Feng*), 1 part
Semen Raphani Sativi (*Lai Fu Zi*), 1 part
Radix Clematidis Chinensis (*Wei Ling Xian*), 1 part
Resina Olibani (*Ru Xiang*), 1 part
Resina Myrrhae (*Mo Yao*), 1 part
Borneolum (*Bing Pian*), ⅛ part

One can then sleep on this pillow every night, placing that part of the head where the pain is the worst on top of the pillow. This formula is for external use only. It is not meant for internal administration. See below for information on ordering Chinese herbs.

Poultices & plasters

Below are a selection of one, two, and three ingredient Chinese herbal poultices and plasters for the treatment of various types

106

of headaches. They are reasonably easy to make, relatively safe, and quite effective. If any of them cause skin irritation or blistering, discontinue their use immediately.

For liver yang headaches, one can take some Fructus Evodiae Rutecarpae (*Wu Zhu Yu*) and grind it into powder. Then mix some of this powder with a little vinegar. Make into a paste and apply to *Yong Quan* (Kidney 1) on the soles of the feet.

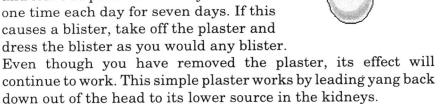

Fix in place with an adhesive bandage and leave in place for one day. Do this one time each day for seven days. If this causes a blister, take off the plaster and dress the blister as you would any blister. Even though you have removed the plaster, its effect will continue to work. This simple plaster works by leading yang back down out of the head to its lower source in the kidneys.

For the first aid treatment of various types of headache, one can mash 20g of white onion. Then grind 20g of Sichuan peppercorns and 12 g of Radix Ligustici Wallichii (*Chuan Xiong*). Mix these together with a little peppermint oil and white flour into flat herbal discs. Apply these discs to *Tai Yang* (Extra channel M-HN-9) and *Bai Hui* (Governing Vessel 20). Hold in place with adhesive bandages or tie in place with cotton gauze. Do this on an as needed basis.

For wind heat headache, take 15g of Excrementum Bombycis (*Can Sha*) and 30g of uncooked Gypsum Fibrosum (*Shi Gao*). Grind these into fine powder and mix with a little vinegar into a paste. Apply this paste to the forehead one time per day. Three to five applications equals one course of therapy.

107

For the first aid relief of headache, take Radix Angelicae Sinensis (*Dang Gui*), 12g, Radix Ligustici Wallichii (*Chuan Xiong*), 6g, and Rhizoma Cyperi Rotundi (*Xiang Fu*), 6g. Grind these into powder and mix with 20g of table salt. Place this powder in a dry wok or pan and stir-fry till hot. Then wrap in clean cotton cloth and apply to the head over the affected area.

For headaches that are characterized by particularly severe wind, grind into powder 45g of Radix Et Rhizoma Notopterygii (*Qiang Huo*) and Radix Angelicae Pubescentis (*Du Huo*), 30g of Radix Rubrus Paeoniae Lactiflorae (*Chi Shao*), 20g of Radix Angelicae Dahuricae (*Bai Zhi*), and 18g of Rhizoma Acori Graminei (*Shi Chang Pu*). Then mix this with the juice pressed from five or more scallions. Make this into a paste and then apply this paste to *Tai Yang* (M-HN-9), *Feng Chi* (Gallbladder 20), and *Feng Fu* (Governing Vessel 16).

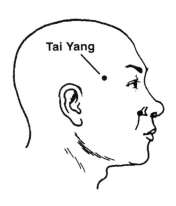

Hold in place with an adhesive bandage. Change one time each day.

One more external remedy for a wind cold pattern headache is to take equal amounts of black pepper and Folium Artemisiae Argyii (*Ai Ye*). Grind these into powder and then mix with a suitable amount of egg white. Apply this paste to *Bai Hui* (Governing Vessel 20) and change this one time each day. Five to seven days equals one course of therapy.

Chinese self-massage

Massage, including self-massage, is a highly developed part of traditional Chinese medicine. The self-massage regime below is specifically designed as a home remedy for headache. For more Chinese self-massage regimes, the reader should see Fan Ya-li's *Chinese Self-massage Therapy: The Easy Way to Health* also published by Blue Poppy Press.

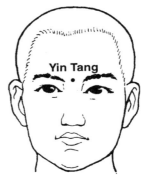

Begin by pressing and kneading the area between the eyebrows above the bridge of the nose. This is the acupuncture point *Yin Tang* (M-HN-3) and is especially useful for calming the spirit and soothing the liver. Do this approximately 100 times.

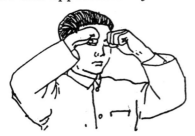

Next, rub the eyebrows with the thumbs and forefingers from the center outward. Do this 100 times.

Third, rub the temples with the tips of the thumbs or middle fingers 100 times until there is a feeling of mild soreness and distention.

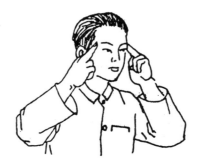

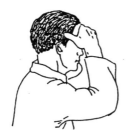

Fourth, rub the temples backward with the edges of the thumbs, from the orbits of the eyes to within the hairline 100 times. Only rub in one direction—from front to back.

109

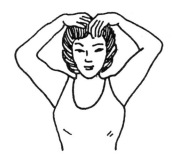

Fifth, place the fingers of one hand on the forehead so that the middle finger is in the middle of the forehead and the other fingers are just below the hairline to either side. The palm of the hand will be resting gently on the top of the head. Now massage backward from the forehead to the center of the top of the head 20-30 times. The hands should move backward by grasping and relaxing the fingertips.

Sixth, pat the top of the head with the hollow of the palm 30-50 times. The point in the middle of the top of the head is called *Bai Hui* (Meeting of Hundreds, Governing Vessel 20). Stimulation of this point calms the spirit and downbears upwardly counterflowing and exuberant liver yang.

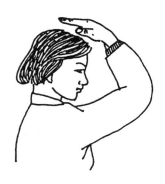

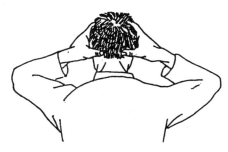

Seventh, press and knead the base of the skull in the depressions on both sides of the back of the neck. This is acupuncture point *Feng Chi* (Gallbladder 20) and is a major point for relieving headache due to upwardly counterflowing liver qi. Do this approximately 100 times.

And lastly, pound the center of the top of one shoulder with the light fist of the opposite hand. This is acupuncture point *Jian Jing* (Gallbladder 21). It also downbears upwardly counter-flowing liver qi. Do this 30-50 times on each side.

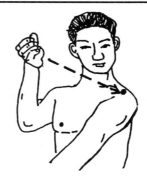

This self-massage regime is appropriate for premenstrual migraines and other types of headaches due to upward counterflow of liver yang or liver fire. It should take between 20 minutes and 1/2 hour. It can be done as a first-aid treatment for a headache currently under way. For chronic, recurrent headaches, one can do this regime once a day or once every other day. In that case, finish by rubbing downward, thumb over thumb the point *Tai Chong* (Liver 3) located in the space between the first and second bones (*i.e.*, the metatarsals) on the top of each foot. This point massaged in this way drains the liver and downbears the qi. Do this 30-50 times.

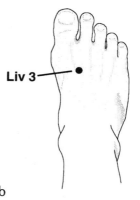

Liv 3

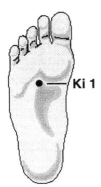

Ki 1

Then knead the point in the hollow of the sole of the foot, just behind and to one side of the ball of the foot: *Yong Quan* (Kidney 1). Do this for 2-3 minutes per foot. This point enriches kidney yin and downbears upward counterflow, therefore using kidney yin to control hyperactive liver yang.

111

Seven star hammering

A seven star hammer is a small hammer or mallet with seven small needles embedded in its head. Nowadays in China, it is often called a skin or dermal needle. It is one of the ways a person can stimulate various acupuncture points without actually inserting a needle into the body. Seven star hammers can be used either for people who are afraid of regular acupuncture, for children, or for those who wish to treat their condition at home. When the points to be stimulated are on the front of the body, this technique can be done by oneself. When they are located on the back of the body, this technique can be done by a family member or friend. This is a very easy technique which does not require any special training or expertise. Seven star hammers (also called plum blossom hammers and dermal needles) can be purchased from:

Oriental Medical Supply Co.
1950 Washington St. Braintree, MA 02184
Tel. 617-331-3370 Orders: 1-800-323-1839 Fax: 617-335-5779

For headache due to invasion of external evils, such as wind cold or wind heat:

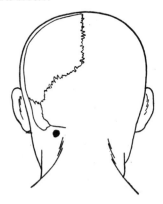

First tap the back of the neck, the upper back, and the region of the head affected by the pain.

In particular, tap *Feng Chi* (Gallbladder 20).

And tap *Tai Yang*
(Extra Channel M-HN-9).

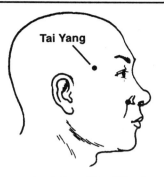

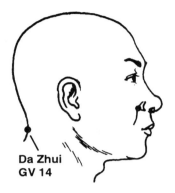

And tap *Da Zhui*
(Governing Vessel 14).

It is ok to tap *Tai Yang* and *Da Zhui* hard enough so that they bleed just a little. If so, clean the area with a sterile cotton ball dipped in alcohol or hydrogen peroxide.

For headache due to internal causes, including liver yang hyperactivity:

First tap the back of the neck and the affected area.

Tap *Tai Yang* (M-HN-9). (See above)

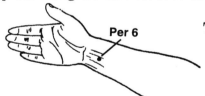

Tap *Nei Guan* (Pericardium 6).

Tap *Wai Guan* (Triple Burner 5).

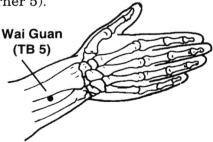

113

Then tap the entire sacrum, all with moderate stimulation. If there is liver fire, tap *Tai Yang* hard enough so that it bleeds just a little. Then clean with cotton and alcohol or hydrogen peroxide as above. In general, one can tap any part of the head where one feels pain.

Between treatments, soak the seven star hammer in alcohol or hydrogen peroxide and do not share hammers between people in order to prevent any infection from one person to another. Seven star hammers are very cheap. So each person can easily afford to have their own. They can also be purchased from Oriental Medical Supply Co. whose address and phone numbers are given in the section on Chinese magnet therapy above.

Thread moxibustion

Thread moxibustion refers to burning extremely tiny cones or "threads" of aged Oriental mugwort directly on top of certain acupuncture points. When done correctly, this is a very simple and effective way of adding yang qi to the body without causing a burn or scar. This method is appropriate primarily for those who suffer from kidney yang vacuity headaches. Those with liver yang hyperactivity or yin vacuity patterns should consult a professional practitioner before using this self-treatment.

To do thread moxa, one must first purchase the finest grade Japanese moxa wool. This is available from:

Oriental Medical Supply Co.
1950 Washington St. Braintree, MA 02184
Tel. 617-331-3370 Orders: 1-800-323-1839 Fax: 617-335-5779

It is listed under the name Gold Direct Moxa. Pinch off a very small amount of this loose moxa wool and roll it lightly between

114

the thumb and forefinger. What you want to wind up with is a very loose, very thin thread of moxa smaller than a grain of rice. It is important that this thread not be too large or too tightly wrapped.

Next, rub a very thin film of Tiger Balm or Temple of Heaven Balm on the point to be moxaed. These are camphored Chinese medical salves which are widely available in North American health food stores or from Mayway Corp. whose address, telephone numbers, and fax numbers are given below. Be sure to apply nothing more than the thinnest film of salve. If such a Chinese medicated salve is not available, then wipe the point with a tiny amount of vegetable oil. Stand the thread of moxa up perpendicularly directly over the point to be moxaed. The oil or balm should provide enough stickiness to make the thread stand on end. Light the tread with a burning incense stick. As the thread burns down towards the skin, you will feel more and more heat. Immediately remove the burning thread when you begin to feel the burning thread go from hot to too hot. *Do not burn yourself.* It is better to pull the thread off too soon than too late. In this case, more is not better than enough. (If you do burn yourself, apply some *Ching Wan Hong* ointment. This is a Chinese burn salve which is available at Chinese apothecaries and from Mayway Corp. It is truly wonderful for treating all sorts of burns. It should be in every home's medicine cabinet.)

Having removed the burning thread and extinguished it between your two fingers, repeat this process again. To make this process go faster and more efficiently, one can roll a number of threads before starting the treatment. Each time the thread burns down close to the skin, pinch it off the skin and extinguish it *before* it starts to burn you. If you do this correctly, your skin will get red and hot to the touch but you will not raise a blister. Because everyone's skin is different, the first time you do this, only start

115

out with three or four threads. Each day, increase this number until you reach nine to 12 threads per treatment.

This treatment is especially effective for women in their late 30s and throughout their 40s whose spleen and kidney yang qi has already become weak and insufficient or in older patients of both sexes. Since this treatment actually adds yang qi to the body, this type of thread moxa fortifies the spleen and invigorates the kidneys, warming yang and boosting the qi. Because the stimuli is not that strong at any given treatment, it must be done every day for a number of days. For women who suffer from PMS with pronounced premenstrual fatigue, loose stools, cold hands and feet, low or no libido, and low back or knee pain accompanied by frequent nighttime urination which tends to be copious and clear, I recommend beginning this moxibustion just before ovulation, around day 10 in the cycle. It should then be repeated every day up through day one of the period and then suspended. It can be done for several months in a row, but should not usually be done continuously throughout the year, day in and day out.

There are three points which should be moxaed using this supplementing technique. These are:

Qi Hai
(Conception Vessel 6)

Guan Yuan
(Conception Vessel 4)

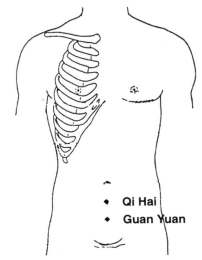

116

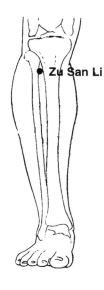

Zu San Li (Stomach 36)

Qi Hai is located on the midline of the body, two finger widths below the navel. *Guan Yuan* is also located on the midline of the lower abdomen, four finger widths below the navel. *Zu San Li* is located four finger widths below the lower edge of the kneecap between the tibia and fibula on the outside edge of the lower leg. However, we *highly* recommend visiting a local professional acupuncturist so that they can teach you how to do this technique safely and effectively and to show you how to locate these three points accurately.

In Chinese medicine, this technique is considered a longevity and health preservation technique. It is great for those people whose yang qi has already begun to decline due to the inevitable aging process. It should not be done by people with ascension of hyperactive liver yang, liver fire, or depressive liver heat. It should also always be done starting from the topmost point and moving downward. This is to prevent leading heat to counterflow upward. If there is any doubt about whether this technique is appropriate for you, please see a professional practitioner for a diagnosis and individualized recommendation.

Chinese medicinal wines

Chinese medicinal wines are part of Chinese dietary therapy. They make use of alcohol's special characteristics as well as a few Chinese herbs or medicinals. Although alcohol is hot and can inflame yang heat, especially liver heat, alcohol moves depressed qi and static blood. It also speeds and increases the medicinal effects of herbs into and within the body. Therefore, one can

117

cautiously make and take a number of simple Chinese medicinal wines for various patterns of headache.

For liver yang hyperactivity causing dizziness, headache, or one-sided headache, soak 200g of Fructus Viticis (*Man Jing Zi*) in one quart or fifth of brandy or vodka for one month. Remove the dregs and drink one ounce or so at the time of the dizziness or headache. A slightly more elaborate formula for the same condition consists of 60g of Fructus Viticis (*Man Jing Zi*) and 30g each of Flos Chrysanthemi Morifolii (*Ju Hua*), Radix Ligustici Wallichii (*Chuan Xiong*), Radix Ledebouriellae Divaricatae (*Fang Feng*), and Herba Menthae Haplocalycis (*Bo He*). Make and take the same way as the preceding "wine."

For depressive liver heat or liver fire with red eyes, headache, and dizziness, soak 125g of Flos Chrysanthemi Morifolii (*Ju Hua*) in one quart of brandy or vodka for one month. Remove the dregs and drink one ounce before or after dinner.

For heart blood-spleen qi vacuity, one can try either of two self-made Chinese medicinal wines. The first is made by placing 150g of white Ginseng (Radix Panacis Ginseng, *Ren Shen*) in one quart or fifth of brandy for 1-2 months. Then remove the dregs, and take 1-2 ounces before or after dinner. However, do not use this wine if you display the signs and symptoms of depressive liver heat affecting the head and face. One can also use 150g of Arillus Euphoriae Longanae (*Long Yan Rou*) steeped in one quart or fifth of sake. In that case, drink 1-2 ounces before or after dinner each evening. Do not take this latter wine if you suffer from constipation.

For headaches due to phlegm blocking or confounding the portals of the heart, take 120g of Rhizoma Acori Graminei (*Shi Chang Pu*) and soak this in one quart or fifth of vodka for 3-5 days. Then

118

take 10-20ml of the resulting medicinal wine three times per day on an empty stomach.

For one-sided headache complicated by either blood vacuity or blood stasis or as a first-aid remedy for any kind of headache, one can try soaking 90g of Radix Ligustici Wallichii (*Chuan Xiong*) in one pint of rice wine for seven days. Drink a small cup each time, two times per day.

These are only a few of the Chinese medicinal wines and elixirs that can be made and used at home for the treatment of headaches. For more information on Chinese medicinal wines, the reader may see my *Chinese Medical Wines & Elixirs* also published by Blue Poppy Press.

Chinese medicinal porridges

Like the Chinese medicinal wines discussed above, Chinese medicinal porridges are a specialized part of Chinese dietary therapy. Because porridges are already in the form of 100° soup, they are a particularly good way of eating otherwise nutritious but nevertheless hard to digest grains. When Chinese medicinals are cooked along with those grains, one has a high-powered but easily assimilable "health food" of the first order.

For wind cold headache, stir-fry till yellow 15g of Fructus Xanthii Sibirici (*Cang Er Zi*). Then boil this in 200ml of water till reduced to 100ml of liquid. Remove the dregs and cook 50g of rice in this herbal "tea" plus another 400ml of water. Eat the resulting porridge two times per day.

For liver fire headache, decoct 200g of uncooked Gypsum Fibrosum (*Shi Gao*) in 300ml of water till the liquid is reduced to 200ml. Remove the dregs and use this to cook 100g of rice plus

119

another 600ml of water into porridge. Eat this every day for breakfast and lunch.

For pain at the top of the head due to liver yang hyperactivity counterflowing upward, cook 50g of rice into porridge with water. When the porridge is half-cooked, add 3g of powdered Fructus Evodiae Rutecarpae (*Wu Zhu Yu*) and cook some more. Towards the end, add two slices of fresh ginger. Eat warm.

For headache associated with high blood pressure in turn due to liver yang hyperactivity, wash 120g of celery and cut the stalks into pieces. Cook with 250g of rice and water into porridge. Add a tiny bit of salt to taste and eat regularly.

For headache in the elderly accompanied by dry, bound stools and constipation, mash 30g each of Semen Pruni Persicae (*Tao Ren*) and pine nuts and 10g of Semen Pruni (*Yu Li Ren*). Boil this mash in water. Then add 30g of rice and cook into porridge. Eat daily on an empty stomach.

For qi vacuity headache, cook 30g of Radix Astragali Membranacei (*Huang Qi*) with 6g of Pericarpium Citri Reticulatae (*Chen Pi*) in 600ml of water for 20 minutes. Remove the dregs and then use the resulting medicinal "tea" to cook 50g of white rice. Another possibility for treating qi vacuity headache is to take 3g of powdered Radix Panacis Ginseng (*Ren Shen*) and cook this with 100g of white rice in water. Yet another option is to take 5g of Ginseng and 20g of powdered Sclerotium Poriae Cocos (*Fu Ling*) and cook this 60g of white rice in water. During the last 5-7 minutes of cooking, add a couple of slices of fresh ginger. If you cannot find Ginseng, you can use 30g of Radix Codonopsitis Pilosulae (*Dang Shen*) cooked with 50g of white rice in water. Remove the Codonopsis at the end and eat the resulting porridge.

For blood vacuity headache, cook 100g of white rice with 15g of Radix Angelicae Sinensis (*Dang Gui*) and 10 red dates (Fructus Zizyphi Jujubae, *Da Zao*). Or cook 100g of white rice in chicken broth plus 10 red dates and eat this for dinner every evening for a number of days.

For headache due to blood and yin vacuity, use 15g of either Semen Biota Orientalis (*Bai Zi Ren*) or Semen Ziziphi Spinosae (*Suan Zao Ren*) with 100g of white rice and again cook with enough water to make a thin porridge or gruel.

For headache due to phlegm confounding or blocking the portals of the head, try cooking 5g of powdered Rhizoma Acori Graminei (*Shi Chang Pu*) with 50g of white rice in water.

For numerous more Chinese medicinal porridge formulas for headaches, see my book, *The Book of Jook, Chinese Medicinal Porridges: A Healthy Alternative to the Typical Western Breakfast* also published by Blue Poppy Press.

Chinese medicinal teas

Chinese medicinal teas may be seen as either Chinese herbal medicine or as Chinese dietary therapy. They consist of using only one or two Chinese herbal medicinals in order to make a tea which is then drunk as one's beverage throughout the day. Such Chinese medicinal teas are usually easier to make and better tasting than multi-ingredient, professionally prescribed decoctions. They can be used as an adjunct to professional prescribed Chinese herbs or as an adjunct to acupuncture or other Chinese therapies for headache.

For wind cold headache, take 9g each of Folium Perillae Frutescentis (*Zi Su Ye*), Radix Et Rhizoma Notopterygii (*Qiang Huo*), and Folium Camelliae Sinensis (*Cha Ye, i.e.,* tea) and grind into powder. Place this powder in a cup and pour in boiling water. Allow to steep for five minutes and then drink.

For wind heat headache, take 6g each of Folium Mori Albi (*Sang Ye*), Flos Chrysanthemi Morifolii (*Ju Hua*), Semen Praeparatus Sojae (*Dan Dou Chi*), and pear skin. Place the herbs in a pot and cover with water. Simmer briefly; then discard the dregs. Drink freely as a tea, one packet per day.

For wind damp headache, take 10g of Herba Elsholtziae Splendentis (*Xiang Ru*), and 5g each of Cortex Magnoliae Officinalis (*Hou Po*) and Semen Dolichoris Lablab (*Bai Bian Dou*). Stir-fry the Dolichos until cooked and pound into pieces. Place the herbs in a thermos and pour in boiling water. Seal the thermos and allow to steep for one hour. Drink freely as a tea, using one packet per day.

For liver yang hyperactivity headache, take 10g of Flos Chrysanthemi Morifolii (*Ju Hua*) and 15g of Semen Cassiae Torae (*Jue Ming Zi*). Place these two ingredients in a cup, pour in boiling water, and allow to steep for five minutes. Drink this freely as a tea, using one packet per day. Another remedy is to use 10g of Spica Prunellae Vulgaris (*Xia Ku Cao*) and 12g of Herba Plantaginis (*Che Qian Cao*). Place these in a cup, pour in boiling water, and allow to steep. Use one packet per day, drinking freely as a tea.

For qi vacuity headache, boil 8g of Radix Panacis Ginseng (*Ren Shen*) for an hour or more in eight ounces of water. Drink this as a tea throughout the day. Asian specialty food stores often sell small porcelian Ginseng cookers. These are lidded cups meant to be placed in a pan of water to create a small double-cooker. Basically, the longer you cook Ginseng, the more you get out of it. As a substitute for Ginseng, you can use double the amount of

122

Radix Codonopsitis Pilosulae (*Dang Shen*). *Do not use Ginseng if you suffer from hypertension or high blood pressure.*

If you suffer from blood vacuity, you can try making a tea from 5-10 pieces of Arillus Euphoriae Longanae (*Long Yan Rou*). Place these dried fruits in a double boiler or pressure cooker and steam thoroughly. Then put them in a teacup and steep in boiling water for 10 minutes. Drink the resulting liquid as a tea. Yet another possibility is to boil 10 pieces of Fructus Zizyphi Jujubae (*Da Zao*) in water until the fruit are thoroughly cooked (*i.e.*, completely soft). Then use the resulting liquid to steep 5g of green tea. Drink this as a tea any time throughout the day.

For yin and blood vacuity headache, boil 15g of Fructus Mori Albi (*Sang Zhen*) in water. Remove the dregs and drink one packet per day. Another option is to grind into powder equal amounts of Fructus Schisandrae Chinensis (*Wu Wei Zi*) and Fructus Lycii Chinensis (*Gou Qi Zi*). Then use 5g of this powder steeped in boiling water for 10 minutes as a tea throughout the day. Or you may use 9g of Semen Zizyphi Spinosae (*Suan Zao Ren*). Pound these into pieces, steep in boiling water for 10 minutes, and drink throughout the day.

For phlegm obstruction, grind Rhizoma Acori Graminei (*Shi Chang Pu*), 6g, Flos Jasmini (*Mo Li Hua*), 6g, and green tea, 10g, into coarse powder. Soak some of this powder in boiling water and drink as a tea any time of the day. (You can also use jasmine tea bought at an Asian specialty food shop.) The doses given are for a one day's supply. Another formula for phlegm obstruction consists of Dens Draconis (*Long Chi*), 10g, and Rhizoma Acori Graminei (*Shi Chang Pu*), 3g. First boil the Dens Draconis in water for 10 minutes. Then add the Rhizoma Acori Graminei and continue boiling for another 10-15 minutes. Remove the dregs and drink any time of the day, 1-2 packets per day.

For blood stasis headache or the first-aid treatment of any kind of headache, you may try boiling 3g of Radix Ligustici Wallichii (*Chuan Xiong*) and 6g of green tea in 300ml of water until only 150ml of liquid is left. Drink this warm either when there is pain or warm before meals, 1-2 packets per day.

For more information on Chinese medicinal teas, see Zong Xiao-fan and Gary Liscum's *Chinese Medicinal Teas: Simple, Proven, Folk Formulas for Common Diseases & Promoting Health* also published by Blue Poppy Press.

The medicinals in all the formulas in this chapter can be purchased by mail from:

China Herb Co.
165 W. Queen Lane
Philadelphia, PA 19144
Tel: 215-843-5864 Fax: 215-849-3338 Orders: 1-800-221-4372

Mayway Corp.
1338 Mandela Parkway
Oakland, CA 94607
Tel: 510-208-3113 Orders: 1-800-2-Mayway
Fax: 510-208-3069 Orders by fax: 1-800-909-2828

Nuherbs Co.
3820 Penniman Ave.
Oakland, CA 94619
Tel. 510-534-4372 Orders: 1-800-233-4307
Fax: 510-534-4384 Orders by fax: 1-800-550-1928

Hydrotherapy

Hydrotherapy means water therapy and is also a part of traditional Chinese medicine. There are numerous different water treatments for helping relieve either stress in general or headaches in particular. First, let's begin with a warm bath. If one takes a warm bath just slightly higher than body temperature for 15-20 minutes, this can free and smooth the flow of qi and blood. In addition, it can calm the spirit and hasten sleep. Taking a warm bath a half hour before going to bed can help insomnia. It can also relieve premenstrual tension and irritability.

However, when using a warm bath, one must be careful not to use water so hot or to stay in the bath so long that sweat breaks out on one's forehead. We lose yang qi as well as body fluids when we sweat. Because "fluids and blood share a common source", excessive sweating can cause problems for women with blood and yin vacuities. Sweating can also worsen yang qi vacuities in people whose spleen and kidneys are weak. Therefore, unless one is given a specific hot bath prescription by their Chinese medical practitioner, I suggest readers not stay in warm baths until they sweat. Although they may feel pleasantly relaxed, they may later feel excessively fatigued or excessively hot and thirsty. The later is especially the case in women who are perimenopausal. In these women, hot baths may increase hot flashes and night sweats.

If, due to depression transforming heat, yang qi is exuberant and counterflowing upward, it may cause migraines and tension headaches, hot flashes, night sweats, painful, red eyes, or even nosebleeds. In this case, one can tread in cold water up to their ankles for 15-20 minutes at a time. One may also soak their hands in cold water. Or they may put cold, wet compresses on the backs of their necks. The first two treatments seek to draw yang qi away from the head to either the lower part of the body or out to the extremities. The third treatment seeks to block and neutralize yang qi from counterflowing upward, congesting in the head and damaging the blood vessels in the head.

125

For those who catch cold easily or who are struggling with obesity, one can use cool baths slightly lower than body temperature for 10 minutes per day. Although this may seem contradictory, since cold is yin and these patients already suffer from a yang insufficiency, this brief and not too extreme exposure to cool water stimulates the body to produce more yang qi. In Chinese medicine, it is not advisable to take cold baths during the menstruation itself as this may retard the free flow of qi and blood and lead to dysmenorrhea or painful menstruation.

Creating a personalized regime

One does not need to do all these home treatments for every case of headache. Rather, one should select several of them as the severity of their disease, time, and personal inclination suggest. If one is already taking care of the Three Free Therapies, it is easy to add Chinese aromatherapy and a choice of Chinese medicinal teas, wines, and/or porridges. Chinese self-massage and seven star hammering are more time-consuming, but they are very effective therapies.

Given the several different Chinese self-therapies in this chapter, no one should be unable to find the materials or the time to put at least one of these into practice. In light cases of infrequent headaches, that may be all it takes. While in more difficult, stubborn cases, one may have to do a couple or three of these to insure a lasting relief from head and face pain.

Chinese Medical Research on Headaches

Below are several typical reports on research done on the Chinese medical treatment of headaches in the People's Republic of China. These have been picked randomly from recent issues of Chinese medical journals published in the People's Republic of China. The first five deal with Chinese herbal medicine. The sixth one deals with acupuncture. And the last one discusses the combined treatment of neurovascular diseases with both acupuncture and Chinese herbs. There are approximately 20 provinces in the People's Republic of China and each province publishes a monthly provincial Chinese medical journal. In addition, each province has a provincial Chinese medical college. Many of these colleges also publish a monthly Chinese medical journal. This means that there are 30 or more Chinese medical journals published each month in China with 40-60 articles per issue of each journal. That means that there are thousands of research reports on the efficacy of Chinese medicine published each year.

As the reader will see, the report below describes what is called a clinical audit. A certain number of patients were given a certain treatment and then they were followed up to see how the treatment worked in terms of the their major complaint. The patients in this study had themselves chosen to be treated with Chinese medicine. In other words, they were not blinded. Likewise, the doctors in this study were fully cognizant of what they were doing. This means that this study was not either single blind or double blind. Likewise, patients' responses were not compared to either a placebo or other comparison treatment. The

127

sole interest in this research was how well a self-selected group of headache sufferers did with a particular Chinese herbal protocol which they knew they were taking and wanted to take.

This is called outcome based research. This type of research mirrors real life practice. It is not an artificial construct seeking to rule out all possible co-factors, such as practitioner and/or patient belief. This type of outcome based research is becoming more and more accepted in the Western scientific community as Western researchers are beginning to understand the limitations and fallacies, not to mention the cost, of prospective, double blind, placebo-controlled research. Such double blind, placebo-controlled research was instituted in the 1960s after the thalidomide disaster and quickly became the so-called gold standard of medical research. However, such research does not mimic real life clinical practice where patients knowingly select their care providers and knowingly select the type of treatment they want, such as standard Western drug therapy, nutritional therapy, acupuncture, or herbal medicine.

As Western researchers move more and more towards outcome based research and away from the cost and artificiality of the double blind, placebo-controlled, prospective study, they will also come to realize that there is a veritable mountain of such outcome based research on the safety and efficacy of Chinese medicine in the Chinese medical journals published over the last 40 years in the People's Republic of China.

"A Report on the Treatment of 86 Cases of Recalcitrant Headache with *Dang Gui Si Ni Tang Jia Jian*" by Jin Shao-xian & Zong Hui-min, appearing in *Tian Jin Zhong Yi (Tianjin Chinese Medicine)*, #6, 1993, p. 8

This clinical audit discusses the treatment of 86 cases of recalcitrant headache with *Dang Gui Si Ni Tang Jia Jian* (Dang

Gui Four Counterflows Decoction with Additions & Subtractions). Of the 86 cases, 74 were out-patients and 12 were hospitalized. Twenty-seven (34%) were men and 59 (66%) were women. Their ages ranged from 12-74 years of age. Nine cases were between 12-20, 26 between 20-30, 18 between 31-40, 21 between 41-50, 7 between 50-60, 4 between 61-70, and 1 case was 74 years old. The course of disease had lasted from a few days to several months in 28 cases, from 1-5 years in 32 cases, from 5-10 years in 21 cases, from 10-20 years in 11 cases, and over 20 years in 4 cases. Western medical diagnosis ruled out that these patients' headaches were due to cervical vertebrae disease, brain tumors, brain abscess, nose or throat cancer, swelling of the eye socket, or retention of inner ear fluid.

Based on Chinese medical pattern discrimination, these patients' headaches were categorized as nothing other than external invasion and internal injury. Their symptoms included hands and feet which were minutely chilly, an ashen white facial color, discharge of chilly sweat, hiccup, vomiting of foamy saliva, and a fine, weak pulse or fine pulse on the verge of stopping. According to Chinese medical pattern discrimination, these signs and symptoms are categorized as blood vacuity cold pattern, static blood obstructing and checking the channels and vessels. According to the author and based on the saying, "If there is free flow there is no pain and if there is pain there is no free flow," this type of recalcitrant headache is due to wind cold evils entering the channels and vessels where they obstruct the clear yang qi. The qi and blood become static and stagnant and this obstructs and checks the vessels and pathways. Thus the qi and blood of the clear portals counterflow chaotically and this produces headache. If evil qi is retained, it may hide for a long time and not be removed. This results in a long course of disease and difficulty curing this condition. The fact that the hands and feet suffer inversion chill and the pulse is fine and on the verge of ceasing clarifies that this disease should mostly be categorized as blood vacuity, cold stasis.

Dang Gui Si Ni Tang Jia Jian consisted of: Radix Angelicae Sinensis (*Dang Gui*), 15g, Herba Asari Cum Radice (*Xi Xin*), 3g, Medulla Tetrapanacis Papyriferi (*Tong Cao*), 6g, Fructus Evodiae Rutecarpae (*Wu Zhu Yu*), 5g, Ramulus Cinnamomi Cassiae (*Gui Zhi*), 10g, Radix Albus Paeoniae Lactiflorae (*Bai Shao*), 12g, mix-fried Radix Glycyrrhizae (*Gan Cao*), 12g, Fructus Zizyphi Jujubae (*Da Zao*), 10g, and uncooked Rhizoma Zingiberis (*Sheng Jiang*), 12g. One packet was given per day during headache attacks. Once the headache was relaxed and resolved, administration was stopped. In between episodes, it is also alright to use double the amount of the above formula made into honey pills. In this case, one can take 10g of such pills 2-3 times per day. If there is repeated occurrence of headache, one can then take this formula as a decoction.

If wind cold was more in amount, then Radix Et Rhizoma Notopterygii (*Qiang Huo*) and Radix Ligustici Wallichii (*Chuan Xiong*) were added. If wind heat was more in amount, Herba Menthae Haplocalycis (*Bo He*), Flos Chrysanthemi Morifolii (*Ju Hua*), and uncooked Gypsum Fibrosum (*Shi Gao*) were added. If wind dampness was more in amount, Rhizoma Atractylodis (*Cang Zhu*) and Radix Angelicae Dahuricae (*Bai Zhi*) were added. If qi vacuity was more in amount, Radix Panacis Ginseng (*Ren Shen*) and Radix Astragali Membranacei (*Huang Qi*) were added. If blood vacuity was more in amount, Radix Polygoni Multiflori (*Shou Wu*) was added and Radix Angelicae Sinensis (*Dang Gui*) and Radix Albus Paeoniae Lactiflorae (*Bai Shao*) were doubled.

If kidney vacuity was more in amount, Fructus Corni Officinalis (*Shan Zhu*), Fructus Lycii Chinensis (*Gou Qi*), and Plastrum Testudinis (*Gui Ban*) were added. If phlegm dampness was more in amount, *Er Chen Tang* (Two Aged [Ingredients] Decoction) was added. If there was liver yang hyperactivity, Cinnamon and Evodia were subtracted and Fructus Gardeniae Jasminoidis (*Zhi Zi*), Radix Gentianae Scabrae (*Long Dan Cao*), Ramulus Uncariae Cum Uncis (*Gou Teng*), and Bombyx Batryticatus (*Tian Chong*) were added.

Of the 86 patients treated with the above protocol, 31 or 36.1% were cured, 29 or 33.7% obviously improved, 21 or 24.5% experienced some improvement, and 5 or 5.7% experienced no improvement. Thus the total effectiveness rate was 94.3%.

Case history: The patient was a 28 year-old, unmarried, cadre who typically had irregular and painful periods. Due to work-related vexation, agitation, and taxation, she became excessively exhausted. She thus developed depression and oppression and an inability to relax, which led to her not being able to fall asleep at night. One week after her period, she experienced dizziness and blurred vision accompanied by piercing pain at the crown of her head which was difficult to bear. She also vomited clear water. After taking some pain-relievers and muscle-relaxants, her pain stopped. One month later, during her period, she got the same headache as before. After this, every month during her period she would get the same headache. Her pulse was fine, weak, and forceless. Her tongue was pale with a thin, white, moist coating. She was given *Dang Gui Si Ni Jia Wu Zhu Yu Sheng Jiang Tang* (Dang Gui Four Counterflows plus Evodia & Uncooked Ginger Decoction): Fructus Evodiae Rutecarpae (*Wu Zhu*), 10g, uncooked Rhizoma Zingiberis (*Sheng Jiang*), 5g, Fructus Zizyphi Jujubae

131

(*Da Zao*), 5g, Ramulus Cinnamomi Cassiae (*Gui Zhi*), 10g, Radix Albus Paeoniae Lactiflorae (*Bai Shao*), 12g, mix-fried Radix Glycyrrhizae (*Gan Cao*), 10g, Herba Asari Cum Radice (*Xi Xin*), 5g, Radix Angelicae Sinensis (*Dang Gui*), 15g, and Medullae Tetrapanacis Papyriferi (*Tong Cao*), 6g. After 30 packets of this formula, there was no further recurrence of the headache and, on follow-up one half year later, the headache had been completely cured.

The Treatment of 52 Cases of Recalcitrant Migraines with *Huo Xue Hua Yu Xiao Tong Tang*" by Wang Xian-qi & Sun Qing, *Xin Zhong Yi (New Chinese Medicine)*, #7, 1996, p. 49

This article reports on the treatment of 52 cases of recalcitrant migraine headache with the self-composed formula, *Huo Xue Hua Yu Xiao Tong Tang* (Quicken the Blood, Transform Stasis & Disperse Pain Decoction). All 52 of these patients had previously taken Western medicine for a long time without being cured. Among them, there were 20 men and 32 women. Their ages ranged from 15 to 55 years old. Five cases were 20 years of age or less, 22 were 21-30, 14 cases were 31-40, seven cases were 41-50, and four cases were over 50 years of age. The shortest course of disease was one year and the longest was 23 years.

Treatment consisted of administering the following formula: Radix Angelicae Sinensis (*Dang Gui*), Radix Bupleuri (*Chai Hu*), Radix Angelicae Dahuricae (*Bai Zhi*), Radix Et Rhizoma Notopterygii (*Qiang Huo*), Radix Ledebouriellae Divaricatae (*Fang Feng*), Radix Ligustici Wallichii (*Chuan Xiong*), 15g @, Semen Pruni Persicae (*Tao Ren*), Flos Carthami Tinctorii (*Hong Hua*), Radix Scutellariae Baicalensis (*Huang Qin*), Rhizoma Coptidis Chinensis (*Huang Lian*), mix-fried Radix Glycyrrhizae

(*Gan Cao*), 10g @. If there was accompanying insomnia, 10g of Semen Zizyphi Spinosae (*Suan Zao Ren*) and 15g of Rhizoma Acori Graminei (*Shi Chang Pu*) were added. The above medicinals were decocted in water two times. Then 500ml of the resulting liquid was drunk warm each time in the morning and evening. Six days equaled one course of therapy. Between each such course, there were two days of rest (when the herbs were not taken). The shortest course of treatment was one course of therapy, while the longest was five courses.

Cure was defined as complete disappearance of all the symptoms with no recurrence on follow-up after one half year. Based on this definition, 36 cases were judged cured. Thirteen cases improved. This meant that their headaches basically disappeared. However, if they became emotionally upset or overworked and fatigued, they did have recurrences. Happily, these recurrences were very slight. Three cases got no effect from the above protocol. This meant that there was no change for the better in their symptoms from before to after treatment with this formula. Therefore, the total effectiveness rate of this protocol was 94.2%.

"Experiences in the Treatment of 36 Cases of Migraines with *Xiong Qi Shao Zhi Tang*" by Huang Cheng-yun, appearing in *Hei Long Jiang Zhong Yi Yao (Heilongjiang Chinese Medicine & Medicinals)*, #5, 1996, p. 32

In this study of 36 cases of migraine headache, 10 patients were men and 26 patients were women. The youngest was 16 and the oldest was 71 years old. Four cases were between 16-20, 16 were 21-30, nine were 31-40, five were 41-50, and 12 cases were over 50 years of age. Twelve cases had been sick for one year or less, 14 cases for 1-2 years, six cases for 3-5 years, and four cases for more than five years. In terms of frequency of attacks, 15 cases had one or more attacks per month, while 21 cases had one or more migraines each year.

Sixteen cases had one-sided headaches, while 12 cases had bilateral head pain. Another eight cases had one-sided and crown of the head pain. Thirty-cases had throbbing pain, five had visual disturbances, 32 had prodromal auras, and 22 had family histories of migraines. Most of the women reported that their headaches had started around puberty.

The treatment consisted of self-composed *Xiong Qi Shao Zhi Tang* (Ligusticum, Pseudoginseng, Peony & Angelica Decoction). This consisted of: Radix Ligustici Wallichii (*Chuan Xiong*), 15g, Radix Albus Paeoniae Lactiflorae (*Bai Shao*), 30g, Radix Angelicae Dahuricae (*Bai Zhi*), 12g, Radix Pseudoginseng (*San Qi*), 6g, Flos Chrysanthemi Morifolii (*Ju Hua*), 10g, Fructus Viticis (*Man Jing Zi*), 10g, uncooked Radix Rehmanniae (*Sheng Di*), 20g, Bombyx Batryticatus (*Jiang Can*), 6g, Lumbricus (*Di Long*), 10g, Radix Glycyrrhizae (*Gan Cao*), 6g. One packet of these medicinals was decocted in water per day and administered warm in divided doses.

In terms of the method for modifying this formula for individual differences, if there was a wind heat pattern, 30g of uncooked Gypsum Fibrosum (*Shi Gao*) and 6g of Folium Bambusae (*Zhu Ye*) were added. If there was a wind cold pattern, 10g of Herba Seu Flos Schizonepetae Tenuifoliae (*Jing Jie Sui*) and 5g of Herba Asari Cum Radice (*Xi Xin*) were added. If there was insomnia, 30g each of uncooked Concha Ostreae (*Mu Li*) and Os Draconis (*Long Gu*) were added as well as 20g of Caulis Polygoni

134

Multiflori (*Ye Jiao Teng*).[11] If there was constipation, then 6-10g of Radix Et Rhizoma Rhei (*Da Huang*) were added. If there was heart vexation and easy anger, 10g @ of Radix Bupleuri (*Chai Hu*) and Radix Scutellariae Baicalensis (*Huang Qin*) were added. If there was nausea and vomiting, 10g of Rhizoma Pinelliae Ternatae (*Ban Xia*) and 12g of Caulis Bambusae In Taeniis (*Zhu Ru*) were added. If there was pain at the crown of the head, 15g of Radix Et Rhizoma Ligustici Sinensis (*Gao Ben*) were added. If there were visual disturbances, 15g of Fructus Lycii Chinensis (*Gou Qi Zi*) were added. And if there was high blood pressure, 12g of Spica Prunellae Vulgaris (*Xia Ku Cao*) and 15g of Radix Achyranthis Bidentatae (*Huai Niu Xi*) were added.

Complete cure was defined as cessation of headache attacks with no recurrence on follow-up after two years. Improvement meant that the number of attacks was markedly decreased and the symptoms were markedly diminished. No cure meant that there was no change in the headaches or that they got worse. Based on these criteria, 24 cases were cured, and 12 cases were improved. Ten cases took a turn for the better within three days, 16 improved within seven, and 10 cases improved within 20 days.

The author of this protocol based the composition of the formula on Ye Tian-shi's statements that, "Initially diseases are in the channels, while enduring disease enters the network vessels since the channels govern the qi and the network vessels govern

---

[11] It is interesting to note that Western researchers are now beginning to understand that curing sleep disorders can have a therapeutic effect on chronic headaches. Chinese medicine treats insomnia quite well without the use of sedatives which cause grogginess the next day. For more information on the Chinese medical diagnosis and treatment of insomnia, see my *Curing Insomnia Naturally with Chinese Medicine*.

the blood. Thus one can know when one must treat the qi and when one must treat the blood." Because migraines tend to be an enduring, long-lasting disease, Dr. Huang feels that the emphasis in their treatment should be on quickening the blood and transforming stasis. However, this formula does also dispel wind, nourish yin, and clear heat. In addition, it includes several medicinals which are known to be antispasmodic, this relieving the spasming of the blood vessels which is associated with migraines.

"An Analysis of the Treatment Efficacy of *Qing Shang Quan Tong Tang* on Vascular Headaches" by Zhang Yue-mei & Fang Dong, *Hei Long Jiang Zhong Yi Yao (Heilongjiang Chinese Medicine & Medicinals)*, #2, 1995, p. 16-17

Between Jan. 1, 1992 and April, 1994, the author of this study treated 34 patients with vascular headaches with *Qing Shang Quan Tong Tang* (Clear the Upper & Purify Pain Decoction). Eight of the patients in this study were men and 26 were women. The youngest was 17 and the oldest was 61. Six were 17-25, 11 were 26-35, nine were 36-45, six were 46-55, and two were over 55 years of age. The shortest course of disease was seven months and the longest was nine years. Eight cases had been ill for one year or less, 16 had been suffering from headaches for 1-5 years, and 10 cases had been suffering for 6-9 years.

Four cases had pain mainly on the left forehead. Six cases had pain mainly on the right forehead. Eleven cases had left-sided temporal pain. Nine cases had right-sided temporal pain. Four cases had bilateral forehead pain. In 25 cases, the pain was throbbing, while in nine cases it was distended pain. Nine cases

136

also had dizziness and vertigo at the time of occurrence, while 17 had nausea and vomiting.

Qing Shang Quan Tong Tang consisted of: Radix Angelicae Sinensis (*Dang Gui*), 12-15g, Radix Ligustici Wallichii (*Chuan Xiong*), 12-15g, Radix Angelicae Dahuricae (*Bai Zhi*), 9-12g, Herba Asari Cum Radice (*Xi Xin*), 2-3g, Radix Et Rhizoma Notopterygii (*Qiang Huo*), 9-12g, Radix Angelicae Pubescentis (*Du Huo*), 9-12g, Fructus Viticis (*Man Jing Zi*), 6-10g, Rhizoma Atractylodis (*Cang Zhu*), 9-12g, Tuber Ophiopogonis Japonici (*Mai Dong*), 10-12g, Radix Scutellariae Baicalensis (*Huang Qin*), 12-15g, Flos Chrysanthemi Morifolii (*Ju Hua*), 12-15g, Radix Ledebouriellae Divaricatae (*Fang Feng*), 9-12g, Radix Glycyrrhizae (*Gan Cao*), 6-9g, uncooked Rhizoma Zingiberis (*Sheng Jiang*), 3 slices.

In terms of individualized modifications, if there was accompanying dizziness and vertigo, 15-24g of Rhizoma Alismatis (*Ze Xie*) and 15-24g of Rhizoma Atractylodis Macrocephalae (*Bai Zhu*) were added. If there was nausea and vomiting, 9-15g of ginger-processed Caulis Bambusae In Taeniis (*Zhu Ru*) and 9-12g of Rhizoma Pinelliae Ternatae (*Ban Xia*) were added. If there was a bitter taste in the mouth, red eyes, and constipation with yellow tongue fur, 9-12g of Radix Et Rhizoma Rhei (*Da Huang*) and 9-12g of Fructus Immaturus Citri Aurantii (*Zhi Shi*) were added. One packet of the above formula was decocted in water and administered each day, with 10 days equaling one course of therapy.

Cure meant that the headaches disappeared and there was no recurrence on follow-up after one year. Marked effect was defined as disappearance of the headaches after treatment, some

137

recurrence on follow-up, but markedly decreased pain and fewer attacks. When these medicinals were given again, they were able to eliminate the headaches. Some effect meant that the aching and pain reduced but were not completely eliminated. No effect meant that there was no change for the better after two courses of therapy. Based on these criteria, 23 cases were cured, seven cases got a marked effect, three cases got some effect, and two cases got no effect. Therefore, the total effectiveness rate was 94.2%.

Case history: The patient was a 38 year-old female who came for her first examination on Feb. 21, 1992. She had had migraine headaches for seven years. She had had several EEGs which were all normal. Doctors at a hospital had diagnosed her as suffering from vascular headaches. She had taken several types of Western medicine but with only very little effect. For the last 10 days, due to work stress, she had been having throbbing, left-sided forehead pain. She complained of photophobia which made her keep her eyes shut and she was afraid to move. The pain was so bad at times, it was difficult to bear, and she could not go to sleep at night. These attacks were accompanied by nausea and vomiting. Her tongue was dark with thin, white fur, while her pulse was bowstring and tight.

Based on the above signs and symptoms, her Chinese medical pattern discrimination was categorized as external wind internally invading. The channel qi, therefore, was inhibited and the network vessels were not freely flowing. The qi and blood was static and stagnant. She was prescribed *Qing Shang Quan Tong Tang* with added flavors (*i.e.*, added ingredients). The prescription read: Radix Angelicae Sinensis (*Dang Gui*), 12g, Radix Ligustici Wallichii (*Chuan Xiong*), 15g, Radix Et Rhizoma

Notopterygii (*Qiang Huo*), 10g, Radix Angelicae Pubescentis (*Du Huo*), 9g, Rhizoma Atractylodis (*Cang Zhu*), 9g, Radix Ledebouriellae Divaricatae (*Fang Feng*), 12g, Herba Asari Cum Radice (*Xi Xin*), 3g, Fructus Viticis (*Man Jing Zi*), 3g, Flos Chrysanthemi Morifolii (*Ju Hua*), 12g, Tuber Ophiopogonis Japonici (*Mai Dong*), 12g, Radix Angelicae Dahuricae (*Bai Zhi*), 10g, Radix Scutellariae Baicalensis (*Huang Qin*), 10g, Radix Glycyrrhizae (*Gan Cao*), 9g, ginger-processed Caulis Bambusae In Taeniis (*Zhu Ru*), 10g, Rhizoma Pinelliae Ternatae (*Ban Xia*), 10g, uncooked Rhizoma Zingiberis (*Sheng Jiang*), 3 slices.

After taking three packets of this formula, the aching and pain had obviously diminished. Hence the same formula was given for another three packets. At the end of that time, all her symptoms had completely disappeared. In order to consolidate the therapeutic effect, another three packets of the same herbs was given. After taking these, she then stopped taking any Chinese medicinals. On follow-up after two years, there had been no recurrence.

"The Treatment of 64 Cases of Static Blood Headache with Self-composed *Zhu Yu Zhi Tong Tang*" by Sun Hai-long *et al.*, appearing in *Hei Long Jiang Zhong Yi Yao* (Heilongjiang Chinese Medicine & Medicinals), #4, 1995, p. 34

The 64 patients described in this study were seen between 1985 and 1993. All suffered from enduring headaches which would not heal, the pain of which felt piercing or stabbing. Their tongues were purple and dark and their pulses were bowstring or fine and choppy. Therefore, all were categorized as suffering from blood stasis pattern headaches. Amongst this group, there were 38 men and 26 women. The oldest was 52 and the youngest was 15 years old. Most of the patients were between 40-50 years of age.

Self-composed *Zhu Yu Zhi Tong Tang* (Dispel Stasis & Stop Pain Decoction) was composed of: Radix Ligustici Wallichii (*Chuan Xiong*), 30g, Radix Salviae Miltiorrhizae (*Dan Shen*), 15g, Semen Pruni Persicae (*Tao Ren*), 10g, Flos Carthami Tinctorii (*Hong Hua*), 10g, Radix Rubrus Paeoniae Lactiflorae (*Chi Shao*), 10g, Radix Pseudoginseng (*San Qi*), 5g, Scolopendra Subspinipes (*Wu Gong*), 2 strips, Rhizoma Acori Graminei (*Shi Chang Pu*), 10g. These were decocted in water and administered, one packet per day, taken warm morning and night.

Complete cure meant that the headaches disappeared. Improvement meant that the head pain diminished, their duration was shorter, and the time between episodes was longer. No effect meant that there was no change in the symptoms of headache. Based on these definitions, 40 cases were judged cured, 22 improved, and only two cases got no effect. Therefore, the total effectiveness rate for this protocol was 96%.

"The Acupuncture Treatment of 65 Cases of Migraines" by Bai Hui-min, appearing in *Tian Jin Zhong Yi Xue Yuan Xue Bao (The Journal of the Tianjin College of Chinese Medicine)*, #2, 1996, p. 17

The author begins by stating that one-sided headache (the term most commonly used for migraines in Chinese medicine) is a type of recurrent vascular headache. It is commonly accompanied by nausea and vomiting. The author of this study has been treating this kind of headache for many years with two acupuncture points. Below is the record of 65 such cases.

140

Twenty-two of the 65 cases or 33.8% were men, while 43 or 66.2% were women. The oldest patient was 57 and the youngest was 15. The longest course of disease was 30 years and the shortest was three months. In 28 cases, the aching and pain occurred on the left side. In 30 cases, it occurred on the right side. And in another seven cases, it was bilateral. CT scan and other modern Western diagnostic methods were used to rule out other diagnoses. During this study, previously used Chinese and Western medications were stopped.

The treatment method consisted of two points: *Feng Chi* (Gallbladder 20) and *Qiu Xu* (Gallbladder 40). After disinfecting the areas to be needled, the needles were inserted at these two points and then manipulated with draining technique. (This is the technique for draining off replete evils.) The needles were then retained for 20 minutes. During this time, they were stimulated two times. One treatment was given every other day, and 10 treatments constituted one course of therapy.

Cure was defined as complete disappearance of all symptoms with no recurrence within one year. Marked effect was defined as a marked improvement in the symptoms. However, there were still slight headaches. Some effect meant that the area affected by the pain was smaller and that the degree of pain was less. No effect meant that there was no improvement from before to after the treatment.

Based on these criteria, 22 cases or 33.8% were cured, 29 cases or 44.6% registered marked effect, 11 cases or 16.9% got some effect, and three cases or 4.6% got no effect. Thus the total effectiveness rate was 95.3%.

Case history: The patient was a 41 year-old woman who worked as an engineering teacher. She was first seen on Sept. 12, 1992. She had had recurrent right-sided headaches for eight years. Often, the attacks occurred when she was overworked or when she was emotionally stressed. When the pain was severe, it was accompanied by ringing in the ears, blurred vision, nausea, and a desire to vomit. She had already tried Western medicine without effect. Neurological examination was negative. X-rays of the vertebrae in her neck and a CT scan of her brain showed no abnormalities. She was, therefore, diagnosed as suffering from migraine headaches.

Treatment consisted of needling the two points of *Feng Chi* and *Qiu Xu*. After the first treatment, the head pain had marked decreased. At night, she no longer had to take sedatives and analgesics in order to go to sleep. After the third treatment, the headache was greatly diminished and extra fatigue from work did not aggravate it. By 10 treatments, the symptoms had all disappeared. Therefore, she was judged cured. On follow-up after one year, her headaches had not returned.

In the author's discussion of this study, they say that one-sided pain is categorized in Chinese medicine as *shao yang* channel head pain. *Feng Chi* and *Qiu Xu* are both points on the foot *shao yang* gallbladder channel. *Feng Chi* is located on the head. It is able to course and free the flow of the channels and network vessels. Further, it dispels wind and stops pain. It is an essential point in the treatment of headache. It is mentioned as a remedy for headache in such early Chinese acupuncture classics as the *Zhen Jiu Jia Yi Jing (The Systematic Classic of Acupuncture & Moxibustion)* and the *Zhen Jiu Da Cheng (The Great Compendium of Acupuncture & Moxibustion)*. *Qiu Xu* is the so-called source point on the gallbladder channel. That means it treats diseases of both the viscera (*i.e.*, liver) and the bowels (*i.e.*, gallbladder). Although it is located on the foot, it is recorded in the *Ling Shu (Spiritual Pivot)* that, "For diseases of the head, choose the foot." (This has since become known as the acupuncture principle of treating points below for diseases above and vice versa.) These two points are combined together based on the principle of choosing points above and below on the affected channel.

"The Treatment of 30 Cases of Neurovascular Headache with Acupuncture & Chinese Herbs" by Li Che-cheng & Xu Hui-min, appearing in *Hei Long Jiang Zhong Yi Yao (Heilongjiang Chinese Medicine & Medicinals)*, #1, 1996, p. 18

Beginning in 1990, the author of this article treated 30 cases of neurovascular headache with a combination of acupuncture and Chinese herbal medicine. Twelve of these patients were men and 18 were women. They ranged in age from 12-61 years old, while their course of disease had lasted from two weeks to 18 years. In 18 cases, headaches had been occurring for more than one year. In most cases, the number of attacks were numerous and frequent. In two case, attacks occurred three times or more each day. In 18 cases, they occurred 1-22 times each day. Another eight cases had headaches one time every two days to one week. While another two cases had headaches one time every 1-2 weeks. In 21 cases, the pain was one-sided, while in nine cases it was bilateral. All the patients were diagnosed by Western medical means as suffering from neurovascular headaches. There was a connection between the occurrence of these headaches and changes in emotions and/or sleep. The pain was mostly very severe and lasted from several minutes to several hours. If the headache was severe, it was typically accompanied by sweating, heart palpitations, nausea, and vomiting.

The Chinese herbal formula consisted of: Radix Angelicae Dahuricae (*Bai Zhi*), 60g, Radix Ligustici Wallichii (*Chuan Xiong*), 30g, Cortex Albizziae Julibrissin (*He Huan Pi*),30g, Radix Glycyrrhizae (*Gan Cao*), 30g. These were ground into fine powder and divided into 20 packets. Each morning and evening, the patients in this study took one packet mixed in water.

The acupuncture consisted of needling *Tai Yang* (Extra channel M-HN-9), *Shuai Gu* (Gallbladder 8), and *Bai Hui* (Governing Vessel 20). Each of these points was needled with even draining/even supplementing hand technique and the needles were retained for 30 minutes. This was done one time each day.

Every person in this study registered a marked effect. After continuous treatment for 3-6 days, either the headaches had disappeared or had decreased in either frequency or duration. Nineteen patients or 63.3% were completely cured. This meant that their symptoms disappeared, their EEG was normal, and that neurological tests were negative. The other 11 cases or 36.7% all improved. Their headaches disappeared. However, if they overworked or experienced emotional tension, they did experience a very slight degree of aching and pain. The authors of this study says that, in their experience, most neurovascular headaches have to do with a combination of wind and blood stasis. Therefore, this treatment aims to dispel wind and stop pain, quicken the blood and move stasis.

144

As stated above, I have abstracted these clinical audits on the effectiveness of Chinese medicine and acupuncture from various Chinese medical journals at random. In other words, I went to my shelf and pulled down a handful of a dozen issues of a couple of different journals and this is what I found. It is only a small fraction of the Chinese research on all types of headaches published in such Chinese journals in the last 40 years.

Personally, when I read these reports, as a clinician, I think they look pretty good. The protocols described did not necessarily cure every single patient, but typically 90% *or more* got some benefit. Those are pretty good odds. If you agree with me, then you might consider trying Chinese medicine and/or acupuncture for your headaches, be they migrainous, tension, cluster, or sinus headaches.

145

Finding a Professional Practitioner of Chinese Medicine

Traditional Chinese medicine is one of the fastest growing holistic health care systems in the West today. At the present time, there are 50 colleges in the United States alone which offer 3-4 year training programs in acupuncture, moxibustion, Chinese herbal medicine, and Chinese medical massage. In addition, many of the graduates of these programs have done postgraduate studies at colleges and hospitals in China, Taiwan, Hong Kong, and Japan. Further, a growing number of trained Oriental medical practitioners have immigrated from China, Japan, and Korea to practice acupuncture and Chinese herbal medicine in the West.

Traditional Chinese medicine, including acupuncture, is a discreet and independent health care profession. It is not simply a technique that can easily be added to the array of techniques of some other health care profession. The study of Chinese medicine, acupuncture, and Chinese herbs is as rigorous as is the study of allopathic, chiropractic, naturopathic, or homeopathic medicine. Previous training in any one of these other systems does not automatically confer competence or knowledge in Chinese medicine. In order to get the full benefits and safety of Chinese medicine, one should seek out professionally trained and credentialed practitioners.

In the United States of America, recognition that acupuncture and Chinese medicine are their own independent professions has led to the creation of the National Commission for the Certification of Acupuncture & Oriental Medicine (NCCAOM). This commission has created and administers a national board examination in both acupuncture and Chinese herbal medicine in order to insure minimum levels of professional competence and safety. Those who pass the acupuncture exam append the letters Dipl. Ac. (Diplomate of Acupuncture) after their names, while those who pass the Chinese herbal exam use the letters Dipl. C.H. (Diplomate of Chinese Herbs). I recommend that persons wishing to experience the benefits of acupuncture and Chinese medicine should seek treatment in the U.S. only from those who are NCCAOM certified.

In addition, in the United States, acupuncture is a legal, independent health care profession in more than half the states. A few other states require acupuncturists to work under the supervision of M.D.s, while in a number of states, acupuncture has yet to receive legal status. In states where acupuncture is licensed and regulated, the names of acupuncture practitioners can be found in the *Yellow Pages* of your local phone book or through contacting your State Department of Health, Board of Medical Examiners, or Department of Regulatory Agencies. In states without licensure, it is doubly important to seek treatment only from NCCAOM diplomates.

When seeking a qualified and knowledgeable practitioner, word of mouth referrals are important. Satisfied patients are the most reliable credential a practitioner can have. It is appropriate to ask the practitioner for references from previous patients treated for the same problem. It is best to work with a practitioner who communicates effectively enough for the patient to feel understood and for the Chinese medical diagnosis and treatment plan to make sense. In all cases, a professional practitioner of Chinese medicine should be able and willing to give a written traditional Chinese diagnosis of the patient's pattern upon request.

For further information regarding the practice of Chinese medicine and acupuncture in the United States and for referrals to local professional associations and practitioners in the United States, prospective patients may contact:

National Commission for the Certification of Acupuncture & Oriental Medicine
P.O. Box 97075
Washington D.C. 20090-7075
Tel: (202) 232-1404 Fax: (202) 462-6157

The National Acupuncture & Oriental Medicine Alliance
14637 Starr Rd., SE
Olalla, WA 98357
Tel: (206) 851-6895 Fax: (206) 728-4841
E mail: 76143.2061@compuserve.com

The American Association of Oriental Medicine
433 Front St.
Catasauqua, PA 18032-2506
Tel: (610) 433-2448 Fax: (610) 433-1832

Learning More About Chinese Medicine

For more information on Chinese medicine in general, see:

The Web That Has No Weaver: Understanding Chinese Medicine by Ted Kaptchuk, Congdon & Weed, NY, 1983. This is the best overall introduction to Chinese medicine for the serious lay reader. It has been a standard since it was first published over a dozen years ago and it has yet to be replaced.

Chinese Secrets of Health & Longevity by Bob Flaws, Sound True, Boulder, CO, 1996. This is a six tape audiocassette course introducing Chinese medicine to laypeople. It covers basic Chinese medical theory, Chinese dietary therapy, Chinese herbal medicine, acupuncture, *qi gong*, *feng shui*, deep relaxation, lifestyle, and more.

Fundamentals of Chinese Medicine by the East Asian Medical Studies Society, Paradigm Publications, Brookline, MA, 1985. This is a more technical introduction and overview of Chinese medicine intended for professional entry level students.

Traditional Medicine in Contemporary China by Nathan Sivin, Center for Chinese Studies, University of Michigan, Ann Arbor, 1987. This book discusses the development of Chinese medicine in China in the last half century.

Imperial Secrets of Health and Longevity by Bob Flaws, Blue Poppy Press, Boulder, CO, 1994. This book includes a section on Chinese dietary therapy and generally introduces the basic concepts of good health according to Chinese medicine.

The Mystery of Longevity by Liu Zheng-cai, Foreign Languages Press, Beijing, 1990. This book is also about general principles and practices promoting good health according to Chinese medicine.

www.acupuncture.com This website is a good place to begin surfing various sites on Chinese medicine and acupuncture on the Web. It provides links to numerous other webpages dealing with these subjects.

For more information on Chinese dietary therapy, see:

The Dao of Healthy Eating: A Simple Guide to Diet According to Traditional Chinese Medicine by Bob Flaws, Blue Poppy Press, Inc., Boulder, CO, 1997. This book is a layperson's primer on Chinese dietary therapy. It includes detailed sections on the clear, bland diet as well as sections on chronic candidiasis and allergies.

The Book of Jook: Chinese Medicinal Porridges, A Healthy Alternative to the Typical Western Breakfast by Bob Flaws, Blue Poppy Press, Inc., Boulder, CO, 1995. This book is specifically about Chinese medicinal porridges made with very simple combinations of Chinese medicinal herbs.

Chinese Medicinal Wines & Elixirs by Bob Flaws, Blue Poppy Press, Inc., Boulder, CO, 1995. This book is a large collection of

152

simple, one, two, and three ingredient Chinese medicinal wines which can be made at home.

Chinese Medicinal Teas: Simple, Proven Folk Formulas for Treating Disease & Promoting Health by Zong Xiao-fan & Gary Liscum, Blue Poppy Press, Inc., Boulder, CO, 1997. Like the above two books, this book is about one, two, and three ingredient Chinese medicinal teas which are easy to make and can be used at home as adjuncts to other, professionally prescribed treatments or for the promotion of health and prevention of disease.

The Tao of Nutrition by Maoshing Ni, Union of Tao and Man, Los Angeles, 1989. This book is also a good overview of Chinese dietary therapy written specifically for a Western lay audience.

Harmony Rules: The Chinese Way of Health Through Food by Gary Butt & Frena Bloomfield, Samuel Weiser, Inc., York Beach, ME, 1985. This book tries to make Chinese dietary therapy more easily understandable for Western lay readers by essentially creating a new system for its discussion. Therefore, its discussion of Chinese dietary therapy is not exactly a standard approach. However, it does include much useful information.

Chinese System of Food Cures: Prevention & Remedies by Henry C. Lu, Sterling Publishing Inc., NY, 1986. This book is somewhat more standard. It includes most of the same information found in *The Tao of Nutrition*. We suggest that you pick one or the other of these.

A Practical English-Chinese Library of Traditional Chinese Medicine: Chinese Medicated Diet ed. by Zhang En-qin, Shanghai

College of Traditional Chinese Medicine Publishing House, Shanghai, 1990. This is a very standard discussion of Chinese dietary therapy written for professional practitioners. However, it is still understandable by non-professional readers.

Eating Your Way to Health —Dietotherapy in Traditional Chinese Medicine by Cai Jing-feng, Foreign Languages Press, Beijing, 1988. This is a slim little book which gives the pith of Chinese dietary therapy. The English is not very good, but the information is certainly ok.

For more information on Chinese patent medicines, see:

Clinical Handbook of Chinese Prepared Medicine by Chun-han Zhu, Paradigm Publications, Brookline, MA, 1989. This book is an excellent reference text for Chinese prepared or so-called patent medicines. It uses a professionally accurate, standard translational terminology similar to that used in this book. So readers of this book should feel comfortable with the terminology in that book. It is beautifully designed and laid out and is easy to use. This is most definitely my first choice of books on Chinese patent medicines.

Outline Guide to Chinese Herbal Patent Medicines in Pill Form by Margaret A. Naeser, Boston Chinese Medicine, Boston, 1990. This book contains basically the same information as the preceding title. However, it is a paperback and is more "home-made" through desk-top publishing. Therefore, it is a cheaper source of essentially the same information in not so nice a package. It also does not use a professionally accurate, standard translational terminology.

For more information on Chinese herbs and formulas, see:

Chinese Herbal Medicine: Materia Medica by Dan Bensky & Andrew Gamble, Eastland Press, Seattle, 1993. This is the "industry standard" when it comes to descriptions of the basic Chinese materia medica. Under each entry you will find the temperature, flavors, channel-enterings, functions, indications, combinations, dosages, and contraindications of all the most important Chinese medicinals, including all the Chinese medicinals mentioned in this book.

Chinese Herbal Medicine: Formulas & Strategies by Dan Bensky & Randall Barolet, Eastland Press, Seattle, 1990. This is the companion volume to the preceding text. It is the industry standard for descriptions of all the main Chinese medicinal formulas. Under each entry, it gives the ingredients and their dosages, functions, indications, dosages and administration of the formula as a whole, and cautions and contraindications of all the most important Chinese formulas, including almost all the formulas mentioned in this book.

Oriental Materia Medica: A Concise Guide by Hong-yen Hsu *et al.*, Oriental Healing Arts Institute, Long Beach, CA, 1986. This book is a pharmacopeia similar to Bensky & Gamble's above. The information it contains under each herb is not as complete, but it contains many more medicinals. Therefore, it is the next place to look when Bensky & Gamble do not list a particular Chinese medicinal you are trying to find out about.

A Clinical Guide to Chinese Herbs and Formulae by Chen Song Yu & Li Fei, Churchill Livingstone, Edinburgh, 1993. This book contains basic information on Chinese herbs as individuals, the

155

main Chinese herbal formulas, and the Chinese herbal treatment of the most common diseases with Chinese herbal medicine. Compared to the above books, this book is essentially meant as a textbook for a *course* on Chinese herbal medicine. In that case, the above books become reference texts for the *practice* of Chinese herbal medicine.

Chinese Herbal Remedies by Albert Y. Leung, Universe Books, NY, 1984. This book is about simple Chinese herbal home remedies.

Legendary Chinese Healing Herbs by Henry C. Lu, Sterling Publishing Inc., NY, 1991. This book is a fun way to begin learning about Chinese herbal medicine. It is full of interesting and entertaining anecdotes about Chinese medicinal herbs.

For more information on Asian insights into psychology & psychotherapy, see:

The Quiet Therapies: Japanese Pathways to Personal Growth, David K. Reynolds, University of Hawaii Press, Honolulu, 1987. This book is a great little introduction to Japanese forms of psychotherapy based on doing, not analyzing. It also talks about the psychotherapeutic benefits of deep relaxation. David Reynolds has since gone on to author a number of other popular books on Asian insights to psychological health, such as *Playing Ball on Running Water* and *Even in Winter the Ice Doesn't Melt*.

Tibetan Buddhist Medicine and Psychiatry: The Diamond Healing, Terry Clifford, Samuel Weiser Inc., York Beach, ME, 1984. This book explains the Tibetan Buddhist approach to the diagnosis and treatment of mental/emotional disorders. Although

Tibetan medicine is not exactly the same as Chinese medicine, they are "kissing cousins" and many of the insights of Tibetan medicine in terms of psychological disorders is very profound and effective.

Chinese Medical Glossary

Chinese medicine is a system unto itself. Its technical terms are uniquely its own and cannot be reduced to the definitions of Western medicine without destroying the very fabric and logic of Chinese medicine. Ultimately, because Chinese medicine was created in the Chinese language, Chinese medicine is best and really only understood in that language. Nevertheless, as Westerners trying to understand Chinese medicine, we must translate the technical terms of Chinese medicine in English words. If some of these technical translations sound at first peculiar and their meaning is not immediately transparent, this is because no equivalent concepts exist in everyday English.

In the past, some Western authors have erroneously translated technical Chinese medical terms using Western medical or at least quasi-scientific words in an attempt to make this system more acceptable to Western audiences. For instance, the words tonify and sedate are commonly seen in the Western Chinese medical literature even though, in the case of sedate, its meaning is 180° opposite to the Chinese understanding of the word *xie*. *Xie* means to drain off something which has pooled and accumulated. That accumulation is seen as something excess which should not be lingering where it is. Because it is accumulating somewhere where it shouldn't, it is impeding and obstructing whatever should be moving to and through that area. The word sedate comes from the Latin word *sedere*, to sit. Therefore, the word sedate means to make something sit still. In English, we get the word sediment from this same root. However, the Chinese *xie* means draining off something which is sitting somewhere erroneously. Therefore, to think that one is going to sedate what is already sitting is a great mistake in understanding the clinical implication and application of this technical term.

Thus, in order to preserve the integrity of this system while still making it intelligible to English language readers, I have appended the following glossary of Chinese medical technical terms. The terms themselves are based on Nigel Wiseman's *English-Chinese Chinese-English Dictionary of Chinese Medicine* published by the Hunan Science & Technology Press in Changsha, Hunan, People's Republic of China in 1995. Dr. Wiseman is, I believe, the greatest Western scholar in terms of the translation of Chinese medicine into English. As a Chinese reader myself, although I often find Wiseman's terms awkward sounding at first, I also think they convey most accurately the Chinese understanding and logic of these terms.

Acquired essence: Essence manufactured out of the surplus of qi and blood in turn created out of the refined essence of food and drink

Acupoints: Those places on the channels and network vessels where qi and blood tend to collect in denser concentrations, and thus those places where the qi and blood in the channels are especially available for manipulation

Acupuncture: The regulation of qi flow by the stimulation of certain points located on the channels and network vessels achieved mainly by the insertion of fine needles into these points

Aromatherapy: Using various scents and smells to treat and prevent disease

Ascendant hyperactivity of liver yang: Upwardly out of control counterflow of liver yang due to insufficient yin to hold it down in the lower part of the body

Blood: The red colored fluid which flows in the vessels and nourishes and constructs the tissues of the body

Blood stasis: Also called dead blood, malign blood, and dry blood, blood stasis is blood which is no longer moving through the vessels as it should. Instead it is precipitated in the vessels like silt in a river. Like silt, it then obstructs the free flow of the blood in the vessels and also impedes the production of new or fresh blood.

Blood vacuity: Insufficient blood manifesting in diminished nourishment, construction, and moistening of body tissues

Bowels: The hollow yang organs of Chinese medicine

Channels: The main routes for the distribution of qi and blood, but mainly qi

Clear: The pure or clear part of food and drink ingested which is then turned into qi and blood

Counterflow: An erroneous flow of qi, usually upward but sometimes horizontally as well

Dampness: A pathological accumulation of body fluids

Decoction: A method of administering Chinese medicinals by boiling these medicinals in water, removing the dregs, and drinking the resulting medicinal liquid

Depression: Stagnation and lack of movement, as in liver depression qi stagnation

Depressive heat: Pathological heat transformed due to qi depression or stagnation

Drain: To drain off or away some pathological qi or substance from where it is replete or excess

Essence: A stored, very potent form of substance and qi, usually yin when compared to yang qi, but can be transformed into yang qi

Five phase theory: An ancient Chinese system of correspondences dividing up all of reality into five phases of development which then mutually engender and check each other according to definite sequences

Hydrotherapy: Using various baths and water applications to treat and prevent disease

Life gate fire: Another name for kidney yang or kidney fire, seen as the ultimate source of yang qi in the body

Magnet therapy: Applying magnets to acupuncture points to treat and prevent disease

Moxibustion: Burning the herb Artemisia Argyium on, over, or near acupuncture points in order to add yang qi, warm cold, or promote the movement of the qi and blood

Network vessels: Small vessels which form a net-like web insuring the flow of qi and blood to all body tissues

161

Phlegm: A pathological accumulation of phlegm or mucus congealed from dampness or body fluids

Qi: Activity, function, that which moves, transforms, defends, restrains, and warms

Portals: Also called orifices, the openings of the sensory organs and the opening of the heart through which the spirit makes contact with the world outside

Qi mechanism: The process of transforming yin substance controlled and promoted by the qi, largely synonymous with the process of digestion

Qi vacuity: Insufficient qi manifesting in diminished movement, transformation, and function

Repletion: Excess or fullness, almost always pathological

Seven star hammer: A small hammer with needles embedded in its head used to stimulate acupoints without actually inserting needles

Spirit: The accumulation of qi in the heart which manifests as consciousness, sensory awareness, and mental-emotional function

Stagnation: Non-movement of the qi, lack of free flow, constraint

Supplement: To add to or augment, as in supplementing the qi, blood, yin, or yang

Turbid: The yin, impure, turbid part of food and drink which is sent downward to be excreted as waste

Vacuity: Emptiness or insufficiency, typically of qi, blood, yin, or yang

Vacuity cold: Obvious signs and symptoms of cold due to a lack or insufficiency of yang qi

Vacuity heat: Heat due to hyperactive yang in turn due to insufficient controlling yin

Vessels: The main routes for the distribution of qi and blood, but mainly blood

Viscera: The solid yin organs of Chinese medicine

Yang: In the body, function, movement, activity, transformation

Yang vacuity: Insufficient warming and transforming function giving rise to symptoms of cold in the body

Yin: In the body, substance and nourishment

Yin vacuity: Insufficient yin substance necessary to nourish, control, and counterbalance yang activity

Bibliography

Chinese language sources

Cheng Dan An Zhen Jiu Xuan Ji (Cheng Dan-an's Selected Acupuncture & Moxibustion Works), ed. by Cheng Wei-fen *et al.*, Shanghai Science & Technology Press, Shanghai, 1986

Chu Zhen Zhi Liao Xue (A Study of Acupuncture Treatment), Li Zhong-yu, Sichuan Science & Technology Press, Chengdu, 1990

Fu Ke Lin Chuan Jing Hua (The Clinical Efflorescence of Gynecology), Wang Bu-ru & Wang Qi-ming, Sichuan Science & Technology Press, Chengdu, 1989

Fu Ke Zheng Zhi (Gynecological Patterns & Treatments), Sun Jiu-ling, Hebei People's Press, 1983

Gu Fang Miao Yong (Ancient Formulas, Wondrous Uses), Chen Bao-ming & Zhao Jin-xi, Science & Technology Popularization Press, Beijing, 1994

Han Ying Chang Yong Yi Xue Ci Hui (Chinese-English Glossary of Commonly Used Medical Terms), Huang Xiao-kai, People's Health & Hygiene Press, Beijing, 1982

Nan Zhi Bing De Liang Fang Miao Fa (Fine Formulas & Wondrous Methods for Difficult to Treat Diseases), Wu Da-zhen & He Xin-qiao, Chinese National Medicine & Medicinal Press, Beijing, 1992

Nei Ke Bing Liang Fang (Internal Medicine Disease Fine Formulas), He Yuan-lin & Jiang Chang-yuan, Yunnan University Press, Zhongqing, 1991

Qi Nan Za Zheng Jing (Carefully Chosen Curious, Difficult, Miscellaneous Diseases), Huang Bing-yuan, Guangdong Science & Technology Press, Guangzhou, 1996

Shang Hai Lao Zhong Yi Jing Yan Xuan Bian (A Selected Compilation of Shanghai Old Doctors' Experiences), Shanghai Science & Technology Press, Shanghai, 1984

Shi Yong Zhen Jiu Tui Na Zhi Liao Xue (A Study of Practical Acupuncture, Moxibustion & Tui Na Treatments), Xia Zhi-ping, Shanghai College of Chinese Medicine Press, Shanghai, 1990

Tan Zheng Lun (Treatise on Phlegm Conditions), Hou Tian-yin & Wang Chun-hua, People's Army Press, Beijing, 1989

Xian Dai Nan Zhi Bing Zhong Yi Zhen Liao Xue (A Study of the Chinese Medical Diagnosis & Treatment of Modern Difficult to Treat Diseases), Wu Jun-yu & Bai Yong-bo, Chinese Medicine Ancient Books Press, Beijing, 1993

"*Xue Guan Shen Jing Xing Tou Tong De Zhong Yi Zhi Liao* (The Chinese Medical Treatment of Neurovascular Headaches," Feng Cun-wei, *Xin Zhong Yi (New Chinese Medicine)*, #9, 1996, p. 39-40

Yi Zong Jin Jian (The Golden Mirror of Ancestral Medicine), Wu Qian *et al.*, People's Health & Hygiene Press, Beijing, 1985

Yu Xue Zheng Zhi (Static Blood Patterns & Treatments), Zhang Xue-wen, Shanxi Science & Technology Press, Xian, 1986

Zhen Jiu Chu Fang Xue (A Study of Acupuncture & Moxibustion Prescriptions), Wang Dai, Beijing Publishing Co., Beijing, 1990

Zhen Jiu Da Cheng (The Great Compendium of Acupuncture & Moxibustion), Yang Ji-zhou, People's Health & Hygiene Press, Beijing, 1983

166

Zhen Jiu Xue (A Study of Acupuncture & Moxibustion), Qiu Mao-liang *et al.*, Shanghai Science & Technology Press, Shanghai, 1985

Zhen Jiu Yi Xue (An Easy Study of Acupuncture & Moxibustion), Li Shou-xian, People's Health & Hygiene Press, Beijing, 1990

Zhong Guo Min Jian Cao Yao Fang (Chinese Folk Herbal Medicinal Formulas), Liu Guang-rui & Liu Shao-lin, Sichuan Science & Technology Press, Chengdu, 1992

Zhong Guo Zhen Jiu Chu Fang Xue (A Study of Chinese Acupuncture & Moxibustion Prescriptions), Xiao Shao-qing, Ningxia People's Press, Yinchuan, 1986

Zhong Guo Zhong Yi Mi Fang Da Quan (A Great Compendium of Chinese National Chinese Medical Secret Formulas), ed. by Hu Zhao-ming, Literary Propagation Publishing Company, Shanghai, 1992

Zhong Yi Bing Yin Bing Ji Xue (A Study of Chinese Medical Disease Causes & Disease Mechanisms), Wu Dun- xu, Shanghai College of TCM Press, Shanghai, 1989

Zhong Yi Fu Ke Zhi Liao Shou Ce (A Handbook of Chinese Medical Gynecological Treatment), Wu Shi-xing & Qi Cheng-lin, Shanxi Science & Technology Press, Xian, 1991

Zhong Yi Hu Li Xue (A Study of Chinese Medical Nursing), Lu Su-ying, People's Health & Hygiene Press, Beijing, 1983

Zhong Yi Lin Chuang Ge Ke (Various Clinical Specialties in Chinese Medicine), Zhang En-qin *et al.*, Shanghai College of TCM Press, Shanghai, 1990

Zhong Yi Ling Yan Fang (Efficacious Chinese Medical Formulas), Lin Bin-zhi, Science & Technology Propagation Press, Beijing, 1991

Zhong Yi Miao Yong Yu Yang Sheng (Chinese Medicine Wonderous Uses & Nourishing Life), Ni Qi-lan, Liberation Army Press, Beijing, 1993

Zhong Yi Nei Ke Lin Chuang Shou Ce (A Clinical Manual of Chinese Medicine Internal Medicine), Xia De-shu, Shanghai Science & Technology Press, Shanghai, 1990

Zhong Yi Nei Ke Xue (A Study of Chinese Medicine Internal Medicine), Zhang Bo-ying *et al.*, Shanghai Science & Technology Press, Shanghai, 1990

English language sources

A Barefoot Doctor's Manual, revised & enlarged edition, Cloudburst Press, Mayne Isle, 1977

A Clinical Guide to Chinese Herbs and Formulae, Cheng Song-yu & Li Fei, Churchill & Livingstone, Edinburgh, 1993

A Clinical Manual of Chinese Herbal Medicine and Acupuncture, Zhou Zhong Ying & Jin Hui De, Churchill Livingstone, Edinburgh, 1997

A Compendium of TCM Patterns & Treatments, Bob Flaws & Daniel Finney, Blue Poppy Press, Boulder, CO, 1996

A Comprehensive Guide to Chinese Herbal Medicine, Chen Ze-lin & Chen Mei-fang, Oriental Healing Arts Institute, Long Beach, CA, 1992

"Acupuncture in the Treatment of Migraine", G. Kukiena, *Fortschritte Der Medezin,* Vol. 103, #25, July 4, 1985, p. 669-672

"Acupuncture in the Treatment of Migraine", Y. K. Batra, *American Journal of Acupuncture,* Vol. 14, #2, June, 1986, p. 135-137

"Acupuncture for Long-term Treatment of Headache in a National Health Center," Y. Y. Sappo Junnila, *American Journal of Acupuncture*, Vol. 14, #4, Dec. 1986, p. 351-353

"Acupuncture in the Prophylactic Treatment of Migraine Headache: A Pilot Study", L. Lenhard & P. M. E. Waite, *New Zealand Medical Journal*, Vol. 96, #738, 1983, p. 663-666

" Acupuncture Vs. Medical Treatment for Migraine and Muscle Tension Headache," L. Loh, P. W. Nathan, G.D. Schott, K. J. Zilkha, *Journal of Neurology, Neurosurgery, & Psychiatry*, Vol. 47, #4, 1984, p. 333-337

A Glossary of Chinese Medical Terms & Acupuncture Points, Nigel Wiseman & Ken Boss, Paradigm Publications, Brookline, MA, 1990

A Handbook of Menstrual Diseases in Chinese Medicine, Bob Flaws, Blue Poppy Press, Boulder, CO, 1997

A Handbook of Differential Diagnosis with Key Signs & Symptoms, Therapeutic Principles, and Guiding Prescriptions, Ou-yang Yi, trans. by C. S. Cheung, Harmonious Sunshine Cultural Center, SF, 1987

Chinese-English Terminology of Traditional Chinese Medicine, Shuai Xue-zhong *et al.*, Hunan Science & Technology Press, Changsha, 1983

Chinese-English Manual of Commonly-used Prescriptions in Traditional Chinese Medicine, Ou Ming, ed., Joint Publishing Co., Ltd., Hong Kong, 1989

Chinese Herbal Medicine: Formulas & Strategies, Dan Bensky & Randall Barolet, Eastland Press, Seattle, 1990

Chinese Herbal Medicine: Materia Medica, Dan Bensky & Andrew Gamble, 2nd, revised edition, Eastland, Press, Seattle, 1993

Chinese Self-massage, The Easy Way to Health, Fan Ya-li, Blue Poppy Press, Boulder, CO, 1996

English-Chinese Chinese-English Dictionary of Chinese Medicine, Nigel Wiseman, Hunan Science & Technology Press, Changsha, 1995

Fundamentals of Chinese Acupuncture, Andrew Ellis, Nigel Wiseman & Ken Boss, Paradigm Publications, Brookline, MA, 1988

Fundamentals of Chinese Medicine, Nigel Wiseman & Andrew Ellis, Paradigm Publications, Brookline, MA, 1985

Handbook of Chinese Herbs and Formulas, Him-che Yeung, self-published, LA, 1985

How to Find Relief from Migraine, Rosemary Dudley & Wade Rowland, Beaufort Books Inc., NYC/Toronto, 1982

Mastering Your Migraine, Peter Evans, E. P. Dutton, NY, 1979

Migraines & Headaches, Understanding, Controlling, and Avoiding the Pain, Marcia Wilkinson, Arco Publishing, NY, 1982

Migraine and Other Headaches, James W. Lance, Charles Scribner's Sons, NY, 1986

Migraine, The Breakthrough Study That Explains What Causes It and How It Can Be Completely Prevented Through Diet, Rodolfo Low, Henry Holt & Co., NY, 1987

Migraine, The Evolution of a Common Disorder, Oliver W. Sacks, University of California Press, Berkeley, 1970

Migraine, The Facts, F. Clifford Rose & M. Gavel, Oxford University Press, NY, 1979

Migraine, Understanding a Common Disorder, Oliver W. Sacks, University of California Press, Berkeley, 1985

Oriental Materia Medica, A Concise Guide, Hong-yen Hsu, Oriental Healing Arts Institute, Long Beach, CA, 1986

Practical Therapeutics of Traditional Chinese Medicine, Yan Wu & Warren Fischer, Paradigm Publications, Brookline, MA, 1997

Practical Traditional Chinese Medicine & Pharmacology: Clinical Experiences, Shang Xian-min *et al.*, New World Press, Beijing, 1990

Practical Traditional Chinese Medicine & Pharmacology: Herbal Formulas, Geng Jun-ying, *et al.*, New World Press, Beijing, 1991

The English-Chinese Encyclopedia of Practical Traditional Chinese Medicine, Vol. 12: Gynecology, Xuan Jia-sheng, ed., Higher Education Press, Beijing, 1990

The Essential Book of Traditional Chinese Medicine, Vol: 2: Clinical Practice, Liu Yan-chi, trans. by Fang Ting-yu & Chen Lai-di, Columbia University Press, NY, 1988

The Foundations of Chinese Medicine, Giovanni Maciocia, Churchill Livingstone, Edinburgh, 1989

The Merck Manual, 15th edition, ed. by Robert Berkow, Merck Sharp & Dohme Research Laboratories, Rahway, NJ, 1987

The Practice of Chinese Medicine, Giovanni Maciocia, Churchill Livingstone, Edinburgh, 1994

The Treatment of Disease in TCM, Volume 1: Diseases of the Head and Face Including Mental / Emotional Disorders, Philippe Sionneau & Lu Gang, Blue Poppy Press, Boulder, CO, 1996

171

Traditional Medicine in Contemporary China, Nathan Sivin, University of Michigan, Ann Arbor, 1987

Zang Fu: The Organ Systems of Traditional Chinese Medicine, 2nd edition, Jeremy Ross, Churchill Livingstone, Edinburgh, 1985

General Index

A

A Clinical Guide to Chinese Herbs and Formulae 155, 168

A Practical English-Chinese Library of Traditional Chinese Medicine 153

a shi points 78-80

abdominal pain, paroxysmal 44

acid regurgitation 44

acquired essence 160

acupoints 160, 162

acupuncture v, 1, 25, 50, 54, 75-78, 80-83, 109-112, 114, 121, 127, 128, 140, 142-145, 147-149, 151, 152, 160, 161, 165-170

acupuncture needles 75, 77, 81

aerobics 93, 94

Agastaches Correct the Qi Pills 60

aging 16, 34, 35, 95, 117

agitation 11, 42, 95, 131

alcohol 3, 34, 77, 86, 88, 89, 92, 113, 114, 117

American Association of Oriental Medicine 149

An Shen Bu Xin Wan 68

Anemarrhena & Phellodendron Rehmannia Pills 68

anger 14, 17, 18, 20, 96, 97, 99, 135

animal foods 90

appetite 20, 41, 43, 66, 74, 99, 100

appetite, poor 41, 43, 66

Aquilaria 103, 104

aromatherapy v, 103-105, 126, 160

Artemisia Argyium 108

aura 47, 49

B

Bai Hui 107, 108, 110, 140, 144

Bai Hui-min 140

Bai Zi Yang Xin Wan 67

Bao He Wan 72

Bao Ji Wan 72

Barolet, Randall 155, 169

belching of putrid gas 44

Bensky, Dan 155, 169

Bi Yan Pian 60

Biota Nourish the Heart Pills 67

birth control pills, oral 3

blockage and obstruction 27, 31

blood 7-12, 14, 17-23, 25, 27-31, 33-37, 43-45, 48-53, 57, 58, 62, 63, 66-68, 71, 72, 75, 76, 78, 81, 83-86, 88-93, 95, 96, 99, 100, 106, 117-121, 123-126, 129, 130, 132, 135, 136, 138, 139, 144, 160-162, 166

Blood Mansion Dispel Stasis Pills 71

blood stasis 28, 31, 36, 44, 45, 53, 57, 71, 72, 81, 106, 119, 124, 139, 144, 160

blood vacuity 30, 31, 37, 43, 45, 48-51, 57, 58, 62, 63, 66, 67, 78, 81, 86, 90, 119, 121, 123, 129, 130, 161

Bloomfield, Frena 153

body, heavy sensation in the 43

bowels 7, 8, 12-15, 22, 23, 59, 81, 143, 161

brain 12, 16, 34, 35, 82, 84, 90, 129, 142

Brain Point 82

breasts, swollen, sore 48

breath, shortness of 43

Bu Zhong Yi Qi Wan 70

Butt, Gary 153

C

Cai Jing-feng 154

channels 7, 19, 22, 23, 25, 26, 33-37, 48, 57, 77, 79, 97, 129, 135, 142, 160, 161

channels and network vessels 7, 23, 33-35, 97, 142, 160

Chen Song Yu 155

175

inhalation therapy 105
Inner Classic 23
insomnia 11, 17, 18, 43, 66, 67, 90, 95, 96, 99, 103, 125, 133-135
insufficiency & weakness 30
internal causes 27, 113
internal damage 33
irritability 42, 48, 62, 80, 96, 99, 103, 104, 125
Jin Gui Shen Qi Wan 70
Jin Shao-xian 128
jue yin 26
Kang Ning Wan 72
Kaptchuk, Ted 151
Kidney 1 107, 111
kidney Qi Pills 70
kidney yang vacuity 43, 57, 69, 114
kidney yin vacuity 42, 45, 57
kidneys 12-17, 19, 20, 33, 42, 53, 81, 84, 88, 107, 116, 125
knee soreness and weakness, low back and 42
Kuei Pi Wan 66

L
Large Intestine 4 78
lateral costal pain 42
Legendary Chinese Healing Herbs 156
Leung, Albert Y. 156
Li Che-cheng 143
Li Fei 155, 168
life gate fire 88, 161
light and/or sound, hypersensitivity to 3
Lignum Aquilariae Agallochae 103, 104
Ligusticum & Tea Mixed Pills 57
Ligusticum, Pseudoginseng, Peony & Angelica Decoction 134
limbs, chilled 43
limbs, heavy 41
Ling Shu 143

lips, pale 43, 90
Liscum, Gary 153
Liu Wei Di Huang Wan 68
Liu Zheng-cai 152
liver 13-18, 21, 22, 26, 28, 29, 33, 34, 36, 37, 42, 43, 45, 48-53, 57, 59, 62-66, 68, 70, 78-81, 84, 88, 89, 93, 96, 97, 99, 101, 105, 107, 109-111, 113, 114, 117-120, 122, 131, 143, 160, 161
Liver 3 78, 111
liver depression qi stagnation 28, 34, 36, 37, 48, 50, 51, 53, 62, 66, 80, 88, 89, 96, 97, 99, 105, 161
liver yang, ascendant hyperactivity of 42, 160
Long Dan Xie Gan Wan 65
low back and knee soreness and weakness 42
Lu, Henry C. 153, 156

M
magnet therapy 114, 161
Magnolia Flower Pills 59
Mayway Corp. 73, 115, 124
menstruation, painful 126
migraine headache 1, 132, 133, 169
migraines v, 1-3, 42, 47, 48, 50, 54, 63, 99, 111, 125, 132-134, 136, 140, 170
migraine, classic 3
migraines, common 3
mixed repletion & vacuity 31
mood 74, 99, 100
Morus & Chrysanthemum Drink 58
Moutan & Gardenia Rambling Pills 63
mouth, bitter taste in the 42, 63, 137
mouth, dry 39, 62
Moxa, Gold Direct 114
moxibustion v, 25, 75, 76, 81, 114, 116, 142, 147, 161, 165-167
moxibustion, thread 114

177

178

OTHER BOOKS ON CHINESE MEDICINE AVAILABLE FROM BLUE POPPY PRESS

3450 Penrose Place, Suite 110, Boulder, CO 80301
For ordering 1-800-487-9296 PH. 303\447-8372 FAX 303\245-8362

A NEW AMERICAN ACUPUNC-TURE by Mark Seem, ISBN 0-936185-44-9

ACUPOINT POCKET REFERENCE ISBN 0-936185-93-7

ACUPUNCTURE AND MOXI-BUSTION FORMULAS & TREATMENTS by Cheng Dan-an, trans. by Wu Ming, ISBN 0-936185-68-6

ACUTE ABDOMINAL SYN-DROMES: Their Diagnosis & Treatment by Combined Chinese-Western Medicine by Alon Marcus, ISBN 0-936185-31-7

AGING & BLOOD STASIS: A New Approach to TCM Geriatrics by Yan De-xin, ISBN 0-936185-63-5

AIDS & ITS TREATMENT ACCORDING TO TRADITIONAL CHINESE MEDICINE by Huang Bing-shan, trans. by Fu-Di & Bob Flaws, ISBN 0-936185-28-7

BETTER BREAST HEALTH NATURALLY with CHINESE MEDICINE by Honora Lee Wolfe & Bob Flaws ISBN 0-936185-90-2

THE BOOK OF JOOK: Chinese Medicinal Porridges, An Alternative to the Typical Western Breakfast by B. Flaws, ISBN0-936185-60-0

CHINESE MEDICAL PALMIS-TRY: Your Health in Your Hand by Zong Xiao-fan & Gary Liscum, ISBN 0-936185-64-3

CHINESE MEDICINAL TEAS: Simple, Proven, Folk Formulas for Common Diseases & Promoting Health by Zong Xiao-fan & Gary Liscum, ISBN 0-936185-76-7

CHINESE MEDICINAL WINES & ELIXIRS by Bob Flaws, ISBN 0-936185-58-9

CHINESE PEDIATRIC MAS-SAGE THERAPY: A Parent's & Practitioner's Guide to the Prevention & Treatment of Childhood Illness by Fan Ya-li, ISBN 0-936185-54-6

CHINESE SELF-MASSAGE THERAPY: The Easy Way to Health by Fan Ya-li ISBN 0-936185-74-0

A COMPENDIUM OF TCM PAT-TERNS & TREATMENTS by Bob Flaws & Daniel Finney, ISBN 0-936185-70-8

CURING ARTHRITIS NATURALLY WITH CHINESE MEDICINE by Douglas Frank & Bob Flaws ISBN 0-936185-87-2

CURING DEPRESSION NATURALLY WITH CHINESE MEDICINE by Rosa Schnyer & Bob Flaws ISBN 0-936185-94-5

CURING HAY FEVER NATURALLY WITH CHINESE MEDICINE by Bob Flaws, ISBN 0-936185-91-0

CURING INSOMNIA NATURALLY WITH CHINESE MEDICINE by Bob Flaws ISBN 0-936185-85-6

CURING PMS NATURALLY WITH CHINESE MEDICINE by Bob Flaws ISBN 0-936185-85-6

THE DAO OF INCREASING LONGEVITY AND CONSERVING ONE'S LIFE by Anna Lin & Bob Flaws, ISBN 0-936185-24-4

THE DIVINE FARMER'S MATERIA MEDICA (*A Translation of the Shen Nong Ben Cao*) by Yang Shou-zhong ISBN 0-936185-96-1

THE DIVINELY RESPONDING CLASSIC: *A Translation of the Shen Ying Jing from Zhen Jiu Da Cheng*, trans. by Yang Shou-zhong & Liu Feng-ting ISBN 0-936185-55-4

DUI YAO: THE ART OF COMBINING CHINESE HERBAL MEDICINALS by Philippe Sionneau ISBN 0-936185-81-3

ENDOMETRIOSIS, INFERTILITY AND TRADITIONAL CHINESE MEDICINE: A Laywoman's Guide by Bob Flaws ISBN 0-936185-14-7

THE ESSENCE OF LIU FENG-WU'S GYNECOLOGY by Liu Feng-wu, translated by Yang Shou-zhong ISBN 0-936185-88-0

EXTRA TREATISES BASED ON INVESTIGATION & INQUIRY: *A Translation of Zhu Dan-xi's Ge Zhi Yu Lun*, by Yang Shou-zhong & Duan Wu-jin, ISBN 0-936185-53-8

FIRE IN THE VALLEY: TCM Diagnosis & Treatment of Vaginal Diseases ISBN 0-936185-25-2

FLESHING OUT THE BONES: The Importance of Case Histories in Chin. Med. trans. by Chip Chace. ISBN 0-936185-30-9

FU QING-ZHU'S GYNECOLOGY trans. by Yang Shou-zhong and Liu Da-wei, ISBN 0-936185-35-X

FULFILLING THE ESSENCE: A *Handbook of Traditional & Contemporary Treatments for Female Infertility* by Bob Flaws, ISBN 0-936185-48-1

GOLDEN NEEDLE WANG LE-TING: A 20th Century Master's Approach to Acupuncture by Yu Hui-chan and Han Fu-ru, trans. by Shuai Xue-zhong,

A HANDBOOK OF TRADITIONAL CHINESE DERMATOLOGY by Liang Jian-hui, trans. by Zhang & Flaws, ISBN 0-936185-07-4

A HANDBOOK OF TRADITIONAL CHINESE GYNECOLOGY by Zhejiang College of TCM, trans. by Zhang Ting-liang, ISBN 0-936185-06-6 (4th edit.)

A HANDBOOK OF MENSTRUAL DISEASES IN CHINESE MEDICINE by Bob Flaws ISBN 0-936185-82-1

A HANDBOOK of TCM PEDIATRICS by Bob Flaws, ISBN 0-936185-72-4

A HANDBOOK OF TCM UROLOGY & MALE SEXUAL DYSFUNCTION by Anna Lin, OMD, ISBN 0-936185-36-8

THE HEART & ESSENCE OF DAN-XI'S METHODS OF TREATMENT by Xu Dan-xi, trans. by Yang, ISBN 0-926185-49-X

THE HEART TRANSMISSION OF MEDICINE by Liu Yi-ren, trans. by Yang Shou-zhong ISBN 0-936185-83-X

HIGHLIGHTS OF ANCIENT ACUPUNCTURE PRESCRIPTIONS trans. by Wolfe & Crescenz ISBN 0-936185-23-6

How to Have A HEALTHY PREG-NANCY, HEALTHY BIRTH with Chinese Medicine by Honora Lee Wolfe, ISBN 0-936185-40-6

HOW TO WRITE A TCM HER-BAL FORMULA: *A Logical Methodology for the Formulation & Administration of Chinese Herbal Medicine in Decoction* by Bob Flaws, ISBN 0-936185-49-X

IMPERIAL SECRETS OF HEALTH & LONGEVITY by Bob Flaws, ISBN 0-936185-51-1

KEEPING YOUR CHILD HEALTHY WITH CHINESE MEDICINE by Bob Flaws, ISBN 0-936185-71-6

Li Dong-yuan's TREATISE ON THE SPLEEN & STOMACH, *A Translation of the Pi Wei Lun* by Yang Shou-zhong & Li Jian-yong, ISBN 0-936185-41-4

LOW BACK PAIN: Care & Prevention with Chinese Medicine by Douglas Frank, ISBN 0-936185-66-X

MASTER HUA'S CLASSIC OF THE CENTRAL VISCERA by Hua Tuo, ISBN 0-936185-43-0

THE MEDICAL I CHING: *Oracle of the Healer Within* by Miki Shima, OMD, ISBN 0-936185-38-4

MANAGING MENOPAUSE NATURALLY with Chinese Medicine by Honora Lee Wolfe ISBN 0-936185-98-8

PAO ZHI: Introduction to Processing Chinese Medicinals to Enhance Their Therapeutic Effect, by Philippe Sionneau, ISBN 0-936185-62-1

PATH OF PREGNANCY, VOL. I, Gestational Disorders by Bob Flaws, ISBN 0-936185-39-2

PATH OF PREGNANCY, Vol. II, Postpartum Diseases by Bob Flaws. ISBN 0-936185-42-2

PEDIATRIC BRONCHITIS: Its Cause, Diagnosis & Treatment According to TCM trans. by Gao Yu-li and Bob Flaws, ISBN 0-936185-26-0

PRINCE WEN HUI'S COOK: Chinese Dietary Therapy by Bob Flaws & Honora Lee Wolfe, ISBN 0-912111-05-4, $12.95 (Published by Paradigm Press)

THE PULSE CLASSIC: A Translation of the *Mai Jing* by Wang Shu-he, trans. by Yang Shou-zhong ISBN 0-936185-75-9

RECENT TCM RESEARCH FROM CHINA, trans. by Charles Chace & Bob Flaws, ISBN 0-936185-56-2

THE SECRET OF CHINESE PULSE DIAGNOSIS by Bob Flaws, ISBN 0-936185-67-8

SEVENTY ESSENTIAL TCM FORMULAS FOR BEGINNERS by Bob Flaws, ISBN 0-936185-59-7

SHAOLIN SECRET FORMULAS for Treatment of External Injuries, by De Chan, ISBN 0-936185-08-2

STATEMENTS OF FACT IN TRADITIONAL CHINESE MEDICINE by Bob Flaws, ISBN 0-936185-52-X,

STICKING TO THE POINT 1: A Rational Methodology for the Step by Step Formulation & Administration of an Acupuncture Treatment by Bob Flaws ISBN 0-936185-17-1

STICKING TO THE POINT 2: A Study of Acupuncture & Moxibustion Formulas and Strategies by Bob Flaws ISBN 0-936185-97-X

THE SYSTEMATIC CLASSIC OF ACUPUNCTURE & MOXI-BUSTION (*Jia Yi Jing*) by Huang-fu Mi, trans. by Yang Shou-zhong & Charles Chace, ISBN 0-936185-29-5

THE TAO OF HEALTHY EATING ACCORDING TO CHINESE MEDICINE by Bob Flaws, ISBN 0-936185-92-9

THE TREATMENT OF DISEASE IN TCM, Vol I: Diseases of the Head & Face Including Mental/Emotional Disorders by Philippe Sionneau & Lü Gang, ISBN 0-936185-69-4

THE TREATMENT OF DISEASE IN TCM, Vol. II: Diseases of the Eyes, Ears, Nose, & Throat by Sionneau & Lü, ISBN 0-936185-69-4

THE TREATMENT OF DISEASE, VOL. III: Diseases of the Mouth, Lips, Tongue, Teeth & Gums, by Sionneau & Lü, ISBN 0-936185-79-1

THE TREATMENT OF DISEASE, VOL IV: Diseases of the Neck, Shoulders, Back, & Limbs, by Philippe Sionneau & Lü Gang, ISBN 0-936185-89-9

THE TREATMENT OF EXTERNAL DISEASES WITH ACUPUNCTURE & MOXIBUSTION by Yan Cui-lan and Zhu Yun-long, ISBN 0-936185-80-5